How to Eat to Beat Your Diet

Unlocking the Secrets to Delicious, Nourishing Indulgence

Brenda F. Dozier

Table of content

Introduction..7

Overview of Conventional Dieting................................11

The Problem with Restrictive Diets.............................13

Embracing a New Approach: Delicious, Nourishing

Indulgence..16

Chapter 1..20

The Science of Satisfying Meals..................................20

Understanding Nutrient Balance..................................23

The Role of Macronutrients in Indulgent Eating..........26

Impact of Flavor on Satisfaction and Satiety...............29

Chapter 2..32

Mindful Eating Techniques...32

Connecting with Hunger and Fullness Cues................35

Slow Eating: A Key to Enjoyable Meals.......................38

Mindful Food Choices for Long-Term Satisfaction.......41

Does eating healthy make you less hungry.................44

Chapter 3..47

Building a Balanced Plate...47

Incorporating Colorful and Nutrient-Dense Foods........50

Portion Control without Deprivation 53

Crafting Meals for Maximum Flavor and Satisfaction 56

Eating to best your diet plan 59

Chapter 4 62

The Psychology of Indulgence...................62

Breaking Free from Guilt and Food Shame...................65

Building a Positive Relationship with Food 68

Treating Yourself: The Importance of Occasional Indulgence...................71

Chapter 5 74

Culinary Creativity: Recipes for Indulgent Eating 74

Flavorful Breakfasts to Kickstart Your Day 77

Satisfying Lunches that Fuel and Delight...................80

Decadent Dinners for Culinary Enjoyment...................83

Irresistible Snacks and Desserts...................86

Chapter 6 89

Dining Out Without Derailing Your Goals...................89

Navigating Restaurant Menus for Indulgent Choices........92

Socializing and Celebrating with Smart Food Choices 95

Tips for Enjoyable and Guilt-Free Eating at Events...........98

Chapter 7 101

Fitness and Fun: Balancing Activity with Indulgence 101

The Role of Exercise in a Balanced Lifestyle 104

Finding Activities, You Enjoy 107

Creating a Sustainable Exercise Routine 110

Chapter 8 113

Overcoming Common Challenges 113

Dealing with Emotional Eating 116

Handling Plateaus and Setbacks 119

Staying Motivated for Long-Term Success 122

Chapter 9 125

Embracing the Journey 125

Celebrating Small Victories 128

Shifting from Dieting to Sustainable Lifestyle Choices ..130

Inspiring Others: Sharing Your Success Story 133

Chapter 10 136

Resources for Continued Success 136

Recommended Books and Cookbooks 139

Online Communities for Support 142

Tools and Apps for Tracking Progress 145

Conclusion 148

Recap of Key Principles...151

Your Personalized Path to Indulgent, Nourishing Eating 154

Introduction

Victoria, resolved to alter her lifestyle, began on a revolutionary adventure with food. Shifting away from restricted diets, she embraced a method focusing on nourishing her body. Prioritizing bright, nutrient-dense foods, Victoria found a wellspring of vitality. The art of making balanced plates and relishing guilt-free, delectable meals became her passion. With portion management as her guidance, Victoria obtained satisfaction without excess. Her culinary ingenuity flourished, allowing her to enjoy luxurious times without compromising her ideals. Breaking free from guilt, she built a joyful connection with eating, and appreciating tiny triumphs. Victoria's experience shows the potential of attentive, satisfying eating—a cornerstone for a lifelong, healthy lifestyle.

In the ever-changing dietary trends and health pursuits, the search for a more sustainable, pleasant, and fulfilling approach to eating frequently feels like traversing a labyrinth of conflicting advice. This is because the landscape is constantly shifting. As a result of the numerous restrictions and stringent standards that are associated with traditional diets, many people are left feeling disillusioned and bored with the quest for a better life. On the other hand, what if there was a paradigm shift, a departure from the normal way of thinking that associates good eating with deprivation? We are pleased to welcome you to a trip that redefines the very essence of how we understand and practice a diet that is both balanced and healthy.

This journey is one in which enjoyment and nourishment come together.

Imagine a situation in which each bite is not only a source of nutrition but also a celebration of flavors, textures, and the pure delight that comes with consuming a meal that has been carefully constructed.

However, this is not about giving in to gluttony or giving up any sense of discipline; rather, it is an investigation into a conscious and satisfying method to nurture both the body and the soul.

The purpose of this investigation is to discover the secrets of scrumptious and nourishing indulgence, with the goal of transforming meals from a mundane routine into a symphony of flavor, health, and gourmet satisfaction.

As we start on this journey, we will first analyze the prevalent standards of restrictive diets, which frequently influence our conceptions of what constitutes healthy living. Understanding the complicated dance of macronutrients and flavor profiles, as well as the tremendous impact that these factors have on our overall sense of contentment, is the focus of our investigation into the science that underpins delicious meals.

Nevertheless, this journey is not limited to the realms of scientific language; rather, it encourages you to embrace the art of mindful eating, which involves cultivating a connection with your body's natural indications for hunger and fullness and relishing the present moment with each mouthful that you take.

Building a balanced plate becomes a gourmet experience, where the canvas is filled with an array of colorful, nutrient-dense foods, and portion management is used as a tool for fulfillment rather than deprivation. Along the way, we explore the psychology of indulgence, discovering the foundations of guilt and shame typically linked to our connection with food. Here, we build a positive mindset that regards occasional indulgence not as deviance but as a necessary component of a sustainable and happy existence.

This journey extends beyond the constraints of your kitchen, providing insights into interpreting restaurant menus, engaging with friends and family, and experiencing life's pleasures without compromising your health goals. It's about finding the delicate balance between fitness and indulgence, knowing that exercise can be a source of joy and life rather than a simple obligation.

As we navigate this path, we address typical challenges head-on, from emotional eating to plateaus and setbacks, offering practical solutions to overcome them and move ahead on your journey to well-being.

 Each chapter is a stepping stone, a revelation, and an invitation to enjoy the entire experience of nourishing your body while relishing the pleasure of each meal.

So, ready to set off on a revolutionary expedition—one that uncovers the secrets to eating not just for survival but for sheer, unadulterated enjoyment? This is not simply a guide; it's an invitation to experience the richness of life through the perspective of nutritious pleasure. Are you ready to begin on a journey where the destination is not a number on a scale but a life loaded with taste, vitality, and the joy of clean living? Let the exploration commence.

Overview of Conventional Dieting

In the world of health and wellness, conventional dieting has long been the cornerstone of our collective drive for healthy living. It's an area painted with promises of quick solutions, drastic transformations, and the attraction of fitting into conventional norms of beauty and fitness. Yet, as we engage in the investigation of this dietary environment, it becomes obvious that conventional dieting generally operates under a paradigm of limitation, restrictions, and a one-size-fits-all approach.

At its foundation, conventional dieting often focuses on a reductionist approach, reducing its focus to a rigid set of rules, caloric limitations, and the elimination of entire food groups. The emphasis, more often than not, is on quantitative indicators rather than the qualitative elements of nutrition. This can inadvertently lead to a mismatch between the joy of eating and the quest for a better lifestyle. In the hunt for a number on the scale, the pleasure obtained from nourishing the body is sometimes eclipsed.

Moreover, the rigid structure of typical diets may unwittingly generate a sensation of deprivation. The removal of specific foods, whether due to calorie limitations or dietary dogma, can stimulate cravings and emotional eating. The psychological toll of continually negotiating the dos and don'ts of a restrictive diet can strain our connection with food, making the quest for health feel like a perpetual war rather than a happy journey.

In the overview of conventional diets, it is vital to note that while these approaches may offer short-term benefits, they typically fall short of delivering a sustainable and joyful path to long-term health. The limitations of a one-size-fits-all strategy become clear as our bodies respond differently to varied nutritional regimens. What works for one individual may not always work for another, underlining the significance of tailored and adaptable approaches to diet.

As we negotiate the nuances of conventional dieting, it is necessary to approach this study with a discerning eye. Recognizing the limitations of severe dietary regimens opens the door to a more holistic concept of health—one that recognizes the delicate interaction of flavour, enjoyment, and nutritional value. This larger viewpoint creates the foundation for our journey towards discovering the secrets to delicious, nutritious pleasure, where the quest for health is not only about the destination but also about loving the trip itself.

The Problem with Restrictive Diets

The appeal of restrictive diets, promising rapid transformations and immediate results, often captivates individuals seeking a road to greater health. However, as we uncover the layers of these diets, the underlying difficulties appear, exposing a complex interchange of physical and psychological challenges. The essence of the situation rests in the fundamental type of restriction—be it caloric, category, or temporal.

Restrictive diets usually place rigorous limits on caloric intake, producing an environment of scarcity that can lead to nutrient shortages. The body, in its wisdom, requires a varied assortment of nutrients to function efficiently. By limiting the variety and quantity of foods ingested, these diets may unwittingly affect the body's capacity to obtain key vitamins, minerals, and other vital components necessary for overall health.

Beyond the physical repercussions, the psychological toll of restrictive diets is similarly important. The implementation of severe standards often generates a distinction between "allowed" and "forbidden" foods. This black-and-white approach can foster an unhealthy relationship with food, generating guilt and humiliation when deviating from the prescribed guidelines. The sheer act of identifying items as off-limits can drive cravings, leading to cycles of emotional eating and, ultimately, derailing the intended health goals.

Moreover, the social consequences of restrictive diets cannot be neglected. The rigorous nature of these regimens can make social gatherings and dining experiences problematic, potentially isolating individuals from the shared delight of communal meals. The sensation of deprivation caused by restricted diets may not only damage one's relationship with food but also influence interpersonal ties, reinforcing the impression that achieving health entails renouncing the pleasures of shared culinary experiences.

While restrictive diets may offer immediate gains, the sustainability of such regimens is generally hampered. The body's adaptive mechanisms can lead to plateaus, diminishing returns, and, in some circumstances, rebound weight gain if normal eating patterns are resumed. The recurrent nature of restriction and relapse can create a depressing loop, weakening the motivation and confidence needed for long-term success.

Recognizing the issues inherent in restrictive diets is a critical step toward a more balanced and sustainable approach to health. As we go through this, it becomes clear that the path to well-being lies not in the extremes of denial but in embracing a holistic understanding of nutrition—one that fosters a positive relationship with food, acknowledges the importance of variety, and allows for the enjoyment of meals without the shackles of stringent rules. This perspective sets the stage for our research of uncovering the secrets of delicious, nutritious indulgence, where health is not a destination but a journey enriched by the harmonious integration of physical and mental well-being.

Embracing a New Approach: Delicious, Nourishing Indulgence

In our pursuit of a better and more meaningful lifestyle, it becomes increasingly obvious that a paradigm change is needed—a departure from the restrictive ideals that typically characterize conventional approaches to dieting. This transition gets us to the center of our journey: embracing a new attitude that transcends the conceptions of deprivation and limitation, inviting us to appreciate the exquisite delights of delicious, nutritious indulgence.

At its root, this new method pivots on the fundamental premise that health and enjoyment are not mutually exclusive. Rather than considering indulgence as an occasional guilty pleasure, we redefine it as a vital and conscious component of our entire well-being. It is a change from the punitive character of traditional diets, a purposeful choice to savory the pleasure of eating while simultaneously sustaining our bodies.

The heart of this philosophy resides in the thoughtful combination of pleasure and nutrition. It's about developing meals that not only satisfy our taste buds but also fulfil our body's nutritional needs. By embracing a varied assortment of foods rich in colour, flavour, and nutrient density, we build a culinary experience that transcends the every day and becomes a source of joy and life.

Crucially, the new method urges us to surrender the notion of banned foods. Instead of categorizing certain gastronomic delights as off-limits, we learn to appreciate them in moderation, savouring the joys they provide without shame or remorse. This adjustment in viewpoint develops a healthy connection with food, converting the act of eating from a source of stress to a celebration of life.

As we engage on this path, it is vital to recognize that sustaining enjoyment is not a license for unbridled excess. Portion control and mindful eating remain guiding principles, ensuring that our culinary choices fit with both enjoyment and nutritional intelligence. This method highlights the intrinsic link between physical and mental well-being, realizing that a satisfied palate contributes to a contented mind.

In our discovery of delicious, nourishing pleasure, we expose a route that not only revitalizes our approach to eating but also redefines our entire relationship with food. It's a change from the rigidity of dieting, urging us to bask in the excitement of flavours, the vibrancy of foods, and the sheer delight that comes with consuming a well-balanced and thoughtfully produced meal. This new approach is not just a departure from the old; it's a welcoming acceptance of a lifestyle where health and indulgence happily coexist, laying the foundation for a more sustainable, pleasant, and fulfilling path ahead.

Chapter 1

The Science of Satisfying Meals

Embarking on the research of the science underlying fulfilling meals uncovers a riveting journey into the intricate intricacies that shape our culinary experiences. Beyond the area of taste preferences, the composition of our meals is an art form impacted by the subtle interaction of macronutrients and the impact of flavors on our physiological and psychological fulfillment.

At the heart of constructing fulfilling meals lies the balance of macronutrients—proteins, fats, and carbohydrates. Proteins, typically considered the building blocks of life, play a critical role in delivering satiety by maintaining blood sugar levels and creating a longer feeling of fullness. Fats, when chosen carefully, contribute to the palatability of meals, improving flavors and aiding in the absorption of fat-soluble vitamins. Carbohydrates, supplied from nutrient-dense whole foods, serve as a key energy source, completing the trifecta of a well-balanced meal.

The science of enjoyable meals dives into the delicate ballet of flavors, emphasizing the enormous impact taste has on our overall contentment. The combination of sweet, salty, sour, bitter, and umami ingredients forms a symphony that not only pleases our taste receptors but also initiates a cascade of sensory messages that influence our experience of satisfaction. Understanding the art of flavor balance allows us to elevate our meals from mere sustenance to a delightful and rewarding experience.

Moreover, the science of satisfying meals extends beyond the immediate pleasures of taste. It involves paying regard to the textures and mouthfeel of foods and understanding the sensory qualities that contribute to our overall happiness. The crunch of fresh vegetables, the suppleness of well-cooked proteins, and the smoothness of particular fats all add layers to the dining experience, making each bite a sensory joy.

In the field of nutrition, portion management emerges as a fundamental part of the science underpinning enjoyable meals. Striking the appropriate balance ensures that we acquire the necessary nutrients without overindulging. This deliberate approach to portioning not only satisfies our physiological demands but also helps us to savor the sensory pleasures of our meals without the weight of excess.

As we navigate the science of satisfying meals, it becomes obvious that the quest for a balanced and full diet is not a compromise but an embrace of both nutritional insight and gourmet enjoyment. It is a journey that intertwines the art and science of nourishment, urging us to experience each meal as a meticulously crafted composition that not only sustains our bodies but raises our total well-being via the gratification of our senses.

Understanding Nutrient Balance

In the search for a wholesome and balanced approach to nutrition, understanding nutritional balance emerges as a cornerstone—an informed and purposeful activity that goes beyond basic calorie tracking. At its foundation, nutrient balancing is about harmonizing the intake of macronutrients and micronutrients to meet the body's nutritional needs, supporting general health and well-being.

Macronutrients, covering proteins, lipids, and carbs, form the cornerstone of nutrient balance. Proteins, renowned as the body's building blocks, play a key role in tissue healing, immunological function, and the creation of important enzymes. Fats, often misconceived, are necessary for energy storage, hormone production, and the absorption of fat-soluble vitamins. Carbohydrates, taken from nutritious grains, fruits, and vegetables, serve as the major fuel for our body, sustaining energy levels throughout the day.

Achieving nutrient balance involves a careful approach to portion sizes and dietary choices. Balancing macronutrients includes examining not just the caloric intake but also the quality of the nutrients taken. Opting for lean proteins, healthy fats, and complex carbs ensures a more comprehensive and sustained nutritional profile, contributing to a sense of fullness and contentment.

In addition to macronutrients, the importance of micronutrients—vitamins and minerals—cannot be emphasized in the pursuit of dietary balance. These micronutrients play a key role in different physiological activities, from fortifying the immune system to supporting bone health. A diet rich in various fruits, vegetables, and whole grains provides the broad variety of micronutrients necessary for optimal health.

Understanding nutrient balance extends beyond particular meals to the overall composition of our daily consumption. Striking a balance between the various macronutrients across meals offers a continuous and prolonged release of energy, reducing the oscillations in blood sugar levels that can contribute to cravings and overeating. This careful approach to nutrient allocation develops a more stable and pleasant connection with food.

As we walk the world of nutrient balance, it is vital to comprehend the individuality of dietary demands. What works for one individual may not necessarily be suitable for another, underlining the significance of tailored and adaptive dietary choices. The solution rests not in rigorous adherence to rigid rules but in creating an understanding of dietary requirements, and making informed decisions that match with individual health goals.

Understanding nutrient balance changes the act of eating into a deliberate and empowering experience. It is a commitment to nourishing the body with the proper quantities of critical components, building a foundation for prolonged energy, vitality, and overall well-being. This approach to nutrition is not a restricted regimen but a conscious and enjoyable journey toward a balanced and harmonious connection with the food we consume.

The Role of Macronutrients in Indulgent Eating

In indulgent eating, where flavor and satisfaction take center stage, a nuanced understanding of the role of macronutrients emerges as a guiding principle. Far beyond mere calorie monitoring, macronutrients—proteins, fats, and carbohydrates—play distinctive and crucial roles in the preparation of delicious meals that not only satisfy the palette but also nourish the body.

Proteins, frequently regarded as the building blocks of life, contribute greatly to the satiety factor in decadent meals. Beyond their structural role in tissues and organs, proteins activate a cascade of signals that produce a lasting feeling of fullness. Incorporating lean proteins into decadent recipes not only boosts their nutritional profile but also offers a more fulfilling and well-balanced culinary experience.

Fats, typically linked with indulgence, are key players in the area of flavor and mouthfeel. Opting for healthy fats, sourced from sources such as avocados, almonds, and olive oil, adds richness and depth to indulgent dishes. These fats contribute to the overall enjoyment of food, making it more palatable without sacrificing nutritious value. The proper use of fats raises sumptuous dining from a brief pleasure to a conscious and healthful experience.

Carbohydrates, often wrongly criticized in certain dietary narratives, are crucial contributors to the sumptuous experience. Complex carbs, sourced from whole grains, legumes, and vegetables, give a steady release of energy, eliminating the spikes and crashes associated with simple sugars. This intentional incorporation of carbs not only contributes to the overall balance of an extravagant meal but also supports prolonged satisfaction and energy levels.

Achieving a harmonic balance of macronutrients in indulgent dining is an art a purposeful and conscientious effort to make meals that are both delightful and nourishing. This method moves the focus from restricted dieting to appreciating the diversity of nutrient-dense foods, building a healthy relationship with indulgent choices that go beyond instant enjoyment.

The synergy of macronutrients in decadent meals is not about restriction or adherence to stringent guidelines. It is an exploration of culinary possibilities, an invitation to experience the complexity of flavors and textures while focusing on the nutritional components that contribute to general well-being. Understanding the varied roles of proteins, fats, and carbs helps consumers to make informed choices, converting indulgent eating from a guilty pleasure to a conscious and satisfying celebration of taste and health.

Impact of Flavour on Satisfaction and Satiety

The impact of flavor on satisfaction and satiety exceeds the domain of mere taste, building a rich narrative that stretches to the very essence of our eating experience. In the complex interaction of our sensory faculties, flavor emerges as a linchpin—a dynamic force that determines not only the pleasure gained from our meals but also our overall sensation of contentment and fullness.

Flavor, typically viewed as a subjective and personal experience, is a synthesis of numerous taste elements: sweet, salty, sour, bitter, and umami. These components not only stimulate our taste senses but also activate a cascade of physiological responses. The perception of a wide and well-balanced array of flavors in a meal is crucial to achieving satisfaction, both hedonically and physically.

In the search for satiety, the importance of flavor extends beyond basic enjoyment to the regulation of human hunger. The brain, intricately related to our taste receptors, gets signals that alter our experience of fullness and contentment. The introduction of a diversity of flavors in a meal not only enhances its palatability but also contributes to a more profound and enduring sensation of satisfaction.

Understanding the impact of flavor on pleasure and satiety gives a roadmap for constructing meals that are not only delicious but also conducive to mindful eating. Bland or monotonous flavors may contribute to a disappointing dining experience, potentially driving overconsumption as the body seeks the enjoyment that diverse and lively flavors may bring.

The combination of natural and whole products, each adding its unique flavor profile, becomes an art—a purposeful effort to produce meals that are not only nutritionally sound but also a source of genuine joy. A well-balanced blend of sweet from fruits, savory from meats, and umami from particular items adds layers to the dining experience, changing it into a pleasurable and holistic affair.

Moreover, the impact of flavor on satisfaction and satiety has substantial consequences for our whole relationship with food. By savoring meals that activate our taste receptors, we establish a favorable association with the act of eating. This thoughtful approach to flavor enjoyment coincides with the greater goal of establishing a healthy and sustainable relationship with food—one where pleasure and nutrients coexist happily.

The analysis of flavor as a catalyst for contentment and satiety pushes us to consider our meals not as a mere means of nourishment but as an opportunity to engage our senses, enjoy diversity, and bask in the joy of wholesome, flavorful eating. It is a reminder that our culinary choices may be both beneficial to the body and a source of enormous joy, producing a tapestry of well-being woven with bright threads of flavor and fulfillment.

Chapter 2

Mindful Eating Techniques

Embracing habits of mindful eating stands as a significant call to remodel our connection with food, transforming the act of consumption into a contemplative and intentional experience. In a world typically marked by the rush and bustle of daily life, the essence of mindful eating is in reconnecting with the present moment and creating a heightened awareness of our relationships with food.

At its root, mindful eating emphasizes a conscious presence throughout meals—a shift from distracted eating habits that usually accompany the fast-paced nature of modern living. By engaging all the senses, from the visual appeal of a well-plated dish to the textures and scents that accompany it, we immerse ourselves totally in the culinary experience. This heightened awareness promotes a better appreciation for the intricacies of each meal.

One important part of mindful eating entails tuning in to the body's hunger and fullness sensations. By creating an affiliation between the physical sensations of hunger and satiety, individuals can detect when to commence and complete a meal. This intuitive approach to eating creates a more balanced and attentive connection with food, minimizing overeating motivated by external cues or emotional reactions.

Chewing food gently and savoring each bite is another cornerstone of mindful eating. This deliberate pace not only enhances the enjoyment obtained from the meal but also allows the digestive system to handle food more efficiently. The act of chewing becomes a mindfulness exercise in itself, generating a sense of gratitude for the nutrients offered by each piece.

Mindful eating also supports a non-judgmental examination of thoughts and emotions surrounding food. By noticing and understanding the triggers that may lead to thoughtless or emotional eating, individuals can create a healthier response to stressors, fostering a more harmonious connection with food and limiting the potential for harmful eating patterns.

Incorporating mindfulness into mealtime routines extends beyond the bounds of the dining table. It entails a careful examination of the origins and journeys of the foods we consume—cultivating an understanding of the work, resources, and procedures involved in delivering nourishment to our plates. This ecological consciousness adds complexity to the act of eating, linking us to the broader ramifications of our dietary choices.

However, mindful eating techniques are a call to rediscover the joy of feeding, one mouthful at a time. By establishing a purposeful awareness of the present moment, tuning into the body's signals, and approaching food with a sense of gratitude, individuals can transform meals into a source of not just sustenance but also profound satisfaction and well-being.

Connecting with Hunger and Fullness Cues

Taking on a journey toward a more mindful and intuitive approach to eating begins with a key element: connecting with hunger and fullness cues. In the cacophony of modern living, when external impulses often influence our eating behaviors, understanding these internal signals emerges as a vital step in building a healthier relationship with food.

The concept of connecting with hunger and fullness cues is upon tapping into the body's intrinsic wisdom—a vital but often overlooked part of our physiological well-being. Hunger, far from being a mere discomfort, serves as a critical warning that our body needs food. By paying attention to subtle cues, such as stomach growls or a soft emptiness, individuals can identify the early signs of hunger and respond to them wisely.

Conversely, acknowledging fullness signs is as crucial. The sensation of fullness communicates that our body has gotten the food it requires, pushing us to complete the meal. This awareness inhibits overeating, allowing individuals to quit when satisfied rather than when external stimuli dictate. Learning to distinguish between physical fullness and the impulse to finish what's on the plate is a cornerstone of this mindful practice.

In the fast-paced rhythm of modern living, it is not uncommon to find ourselves separated from these natural signs. The discipline of connecting with hunger and fullness entails slowing down, both physically and emotionally, throughout meals. Taking conscious pauses between meals and assessing the growing feelings within the body builds a more attentive interaction with these cues.

Mindful eating also urges individuals to abandon the notion of "good" or "bad" foods and instead focus on the nutrients and satisfaction each meal delivers. This shift in perspective allows for a more honest connection with the body's signals, enabling individuals to make choices based on genuine hunger and satisfaction rather than external pressures or emotional responses.

Cultivating the art of connecting with hunger and fullness cues is not about enforcing rigid rules but rather about fostering a conscious and intuitive awareness of the body's demands. It is a continuous activity that enables individuals to recover control over their eating patterns, encouraging a balanced and happy relationship with food. By recognizing hunger and fullness as helpful guides, individuals can embark on a journey toward a more fulfilling, sustainable, and nourishing approach to eating.

Slow Eating: A Key to Enjoyable Meals

In the hectic terrain of modern life, where time seems to be an elusive commodity, the practice of slow eating emerges as a significant yet frequently ignored art—a means to transforming meals into joyful and attentive experiences. At its foundation, slow eating is not simply a pace; it's a purposeful approach that encourages folks to savor each mouthful, building a deeper connection with the act of eating and the sustenance it delivers.

The concept of leisurely eating relies upon the awareness that meals are more than a basic replenishment ritual. It is a purposeful act of carving out a place in our hectic schedules to engage with our meals thoroughly. By slowing down the speed of eating, individuals create an environment where every mouthful is a time of sensory exploration, an opportunity to absorb flavors, textures, and scents.

The benefits of deliberate dining extend beyond the initial enjoyment of a well-crafted meal. Research suggests that eating at a more leisurely pace permits the body's natural satiety signals to function efficiently. By giving the digestive system adequate time to absorb each meal, individuals are more likely to identify feelings of fullness, reducing overeating and establishing a healthier connection with food.

Moreover, the practice of leisurely eating develops a careful approach to portion control. By paying attention to the body's signs and eating with heightened awareness, individuals are more equipped to discriminate between actual hunger and external influences, making more educated choices about when to start and stop eating. This intentional interaction with portion sizes contributes to the overall happiness and satisfaction obtained from meals.

In the context of the social and cultural significance of shared meals, unhurried eating also develops a stronger connection with our surroundings and fellow diners. It transforms the act of dining into a community experience, fostering conversations and the appreciation of the shared gastronomic journey. This planned approach to group meals not only nourishes the body but also deepens the links of human connection.

Slow eating, rather than being a hard set of rules, is a flexible and adaptable habit that can be implemented into varied lives. It invites individuals to reclaim a sense of agency over their eating patterns, creating a balanced and happy relationship with food. As we embrace the art of slow eating, we learn that the act of sustenance is not simply a means to a goal but a sensory and social experience, an opportunity to relish the richness of life, one bite at a time.

Mindful Food Choices for Long-Term Satisfaction

In the maze of nutritional choices, the concept of mindful eating choices stands as a compass—a guiding principle for people seeking not just temporary gratification but a persistent sense of well-being. Mindful eating choices transcend beyond the world of calorie monitoring or restrictive diets; they are anchored in a purposeful and intentional approach to sustenance that reverberates in the body's vitality and long-term satisfaction.

At the heart of mindful eating choices lies an understanding of the underlying relationship between the food we consume and its impact on our overall health. It transcends the binary of "good" and "bad" foods, urging individuals to evaluate the nutritional worth and the broader consequences of their dietary selections. This sensitive approach generates a sense of empowerment, allowing individuals to choose choices that match their health goals while still enjoying a varied and fulfilling diet.

Mindful meal choices also emphasize the necessity of listening to the body's messages. Rather than succumbing to external cues or emotional impulses, persons trained to mindful eating pay attention to hunger and fullness cues.

This approach not only reduces overeating but also develops a more intuitive and sustainable connection with food—one where meals are enjoyed in response to true physical demands rather than external constraints.

In the goal of long-term satisfaction, thoughtful meal choices extend to the quality and source of the foods selected. Opting for full, nutrient-dense foods over processed alternatives promotes a balanced and varied dietary intake. Incorporating a diverse assortment of fruits, vegetables, lean proteins, and whole grains not only contributes to general health but also adds brightness and delight to meals.

Cultivating a thoughtful attitude to food choices also entails an appreciation of the greater context of eating. This includes examining the environmental impact of food production, supporting local and sustainable practices, and acknowledging the interconnectedness of our dietary choices with the well-being of the earth. This holistic viewpoint adds complexity to the act of eating, integrating our personal decisions with a greater ethos of health and sustainability.

Mindful eating choices are not about harsh rules or deprivation but about fostering a conscious and harmonious relationship with the meals we consume. It is an invitation to savor each bite, to appreciate the complexity of aromas and textures, and to derive satisfaction not just from the immediate pleasure of eating but from the long-term advantages of nourishing the body. Through mindful food choices, individuals start on a journey of wellness—one that appreciates the art of eating as a source of both joy and lasting vitality.

Does eating healthy make you less hungry

Eating well is generally associated with a plethora of benefits, one of which is the potential to regulate hunger more successfully. While it may seem paradoxical, adopting a balanced and healthy diet can indeed contribute to a reduction in sensations of hunger. Let's study how this complicated interaction between healthy eating and hunger unfolds.

Whole, nutrient-dense foods, such as fruits, vegetables, lean proteins, and whole grains, form the cornerstone of a balanced diet. These meals are rich in critical nutrients, fiber, and satiating components that produce a sense of fullness and contentment. Unlike processed foods which are often high in empty calories and low in nutritional content, whole foods give a constant and prolonged release of energy, helping to suppress frequent hunger pains.

Fiber, in particular, plays a critical function in producing a feeling of fullness. It not only adds heft to your meals but also slows down the digestion process. This leads to a steadier release of nutrients into the bloodstream, reducing fast spikes and dips in blood sugar levels, which can cause hunger. Foods like legumes, whole grains, and veggies are excellent sources of fiber that lead to lasting satiety.

In addition to fiber, the balanced combination of macronutrients - proteins, lipids, and carbs – in a healthy diet adds to greater pleasure after meals. Proteins, renowned for their function in muscle repair and maintenance, are also extremely satiating. Including appropriate protein in your meals will help you feel fuller for a more extended period, lowering the frequency of between-meal cravings.

Healthy fats, coming from foods like avocados, almonds, and olive oil, contribute to the overall sensory experience of meals. The richness and flavor supplied by these fats add to the satisfaction of eating, making you less likely to crave more snacks quickly after a meal.

Moreover, adopting healthy eating habits generally entails attentive and intentional choices. Practicing mindfulness during meals creates a stronger connection with your body's hunger and fullness indicators. When you pay attention to the sensory parts of eating — the flavors, textures, and scents – you tend to enjoy your food more thoroughly, and this satisfaction might translate into feeling less hungry between meals.

It's crucial to note that individual responses to food might vary, and factors such as metabolism, physical activity, and overall health have significant effects. While good food can lead to reduced hunger, it's equally vital to listen to your body's signals and make modifications based on your particular needs.

Adopting a healthy and balanced diet might certainly have a favorable impact on your hunger levels. The combination of nutrient-dense foods, fiber, balanced macronutrients, and mindful eating practices contributes to a more fulfilling and nourishing culinary experience, ultimately improving your overall well-being.

Chapter 3

Building a Balanced Plate

Constructing a balanced plate is a culinary art that exceeds the limits of ordinary food; it is a symphony of flavors, textures, and nutrients that contribute to both delight and well-being. This purposeful approach to meal composition serves as a cornerstone of mindful eating, enabling individuals to build plates that harmonize nutritional intelligence with the delights of the palette.

At the center of a balanced meal lies a smart allocation of macronutrients proteins, lipids, and carbohydrates. Proteins, frequently praised as the building blocks of life, play a key role in tissue healing and the manufacture of critical enzymes. Selecting lean protein sources, such as poultry, fish, or lentils, provides a substantive and fulfilling aspect to the menu while meeting the body's core needs.

Healthy fats, carefully picked from sources like avocados, almonds, and olive oil, not only enhance the palatability of a meal but also add to a sensation of satiety. These fats play a critical function in food absorption, giving a flavorful dimension to the dining experience without compromising on nutritional content.

Completing the trifecta of macronutrients are carbs, acquired from whole grains, fruits, and vegetables. These complex carbs provide continuous energy, eliminating the spikes and crashes associated with refined sugars. Balancing the plate with an adequate amount of carbs ensures a consistent and durable supply of vitality.

Beyond macronutrients, the brilliant colors on the plate symbolize a vast assortment of vitamins, minerals, and antioxidants. The visual diversity of fruits and vegetables not only offers an aesthetic appeal but also represents a vast spectrum of nutrients needed for maintaining optimal health. This infusion of color is a testimonial to the nutritious value of the meal.

Portion control, a vital component of producing a balanced plate, is an exercise in mindful eating. Striking the appropriate balance ensures that the body receives the necessary nutrition without overindulging. This mindful approach to portioning helps both physiological well-being and the enjoyment of the culinary experience.

Making a balanced meal is an elegant blend of nutritional science and sensual enjoyment. It is an invitation to embrace each meal as a symphony of tastes and sensations, supporting both satisfaction and prolonged health. By adopting the principles of balance, diversity, and mindfulness, individuals begin on a path of gastronomic enjoyment that corresponds with their greater wellness goals.

Incorporating Colourful and Nutrient-Dense Foods

The combination of colorful and nutrient-dense foods stands as a brilliant testament to the art of mindful eating—an act that not only pleases the senses but nourishes the body with an assortment of necessary nutrients. This intentional infusion of hues on the dish is more than a visual extravaganza; it is a strategic move toward boosting health and well-being.

The rich and varied colors present in fruits and vegetables are indicative of the vast assortment of vitamins, minerals, and antioxidants they house. These natural substances have key functions in strengthening the body's immune system, eliminating free radicals, and promoting overall health. By adopting a multitude of colors, folks not only raise the visual attractiveness of their meals but also enrich their nutritional profile.

The concept of nutrient density further highlights the necessity of picking foods that carry a nutritional punch. Dark leafy greens, vivid berries, and richly colorful veggies are loaded with important elements, delivering a smorgasbord of health advantages. These foods contribute to a well-balanced diet by supplying a spectrum of vitamins, minerals, and phytochemicals needed for proper physiological functioning.

Beyond the visual attractiveness, adopting colorful and nutrient-dense foods offers a practical strategy for reaching dietary goals. By expanding the palette, individuals are more likely to consume a broader spectrum of nutrients, ensuring that their nutritional demands are addressed fully and holistically. This mindful approach to food choices fosters a sense of vigor and supports long-term health goals.

The practice of including a rainbow of colors on the plate is not bound to the confines of specific diets or restrictions. It is a flexible and fun method that can be tailored to varied culinary preferences and cultural backgrounds. Whether through brilliant salads, juicy fruit bowls, or artfully constructed veggie dishes, the integration of colorful foods is an invitation to savor the richness of flavor while feeding the body with important nutrients.

Enjoying the vibrancy of colorful and nutrient-dense foods is an ode to the synergy of health and gourmet delight. It is a celebration of the numerous and wonderful offers that nature provides, elevating the act of eating to a wholesome and joyful experience. By infusing a range of colors into meals, individuals begin on a journey toward not only visual and gastronomic pleasure but also prolonged well-being.

Portion Control without Deprivation

Mastering the art of portion management is not a punitive exercise; it is a subtle talent that allows individuals to savor the pleasures of eating while maintaining a balanced and healthful lifestyle. It is an invitation to taste the delights of gastronomic encounters without succumbing to the traps of overindulgence, finding a perfect balance that nurtures both satisfaction and well-being.

Portion management is not synonymous with deprivation. Instead, it is a careful and measured approach to managing food intake. By paying attention to portion proportions, consumers can enjoy a varied selection of foods without feeling constrained. This approach develops a focused awareness of the flavors and textures present in each meal, increasing the entire dining experience.

One successful technique for portion control entails listening to the body's hunger and fullness sensations. By tuning in to these signals, individuals can identify when to begin and stop a meal, preventing the normal tendency to eat past satiety. This intuitive method develops a balanced connection with food, grounded in a true response to the body's needs rather than extrinsic stimuli.

Another component of portion management is the strategic distribution of macronutrients on the plate. Balancing proteins, fats, and carbohydrates produces a well-rounded and fulfilling dinner. Proteins contribute to satiety, lipids offer flavor and depth, while carbohydrates provide sustained energy. This careful composition not only supports nutritional goals but also leads to a more satisfying dining experience.

The role of awareness extends to the pace of eating. Eating deliberately and savoring each meal assists the body to sense fullness more efficiently. This methodical pace fosters a sense of enjoyment and satiety, lowering the likelihood of overeating prompted by external cues or distractions. It transforms the act of eating into a focused and enjoyable ritual.

Portion management is not about following tight rules or severe limits; it is a flexible and adaptive discipline that can be implemented into varied lives. It empowers individuals to make informed decisions about the quantity and quality of their food intake, ensuring that each meal is both satisfying and linked with greater health goals. By mastering portion management without deprivation, individuals embark on a

path toward a balanced and sustainable attitude to eating—
one where pleasure and well-being coexist happily.

Crafting Meals for Maximum Flavor and Satisfaction

Crafting meals for maximum flavor and enjoyment is a culinary pursuit that not only tantalizes the taste buds but also pleasingly nourishes the body. This intentional approach to meal preparation transforms eating into an experience that exceeds plain nutrition, raising it to a celebration of different flavors and textures.

One element to getting maximum flavor is the judicious use of herbs and spices. These fragrant additions not only enhance the taste of dishes but also bring unique health advantages. From the anti-inflammatory characteristics of turmeric to the antioxidant-rich nature of herbs like rosemary and thyme, combining a range of spices into meals is a delectable and beneficial endeavor.

Balancing sweet, salty, sour, bitter, and umami sensations creates a symphony of tastes that captivates the mouth. Utilizing elements such as citrus fruits, vinegar, and fermented foods offers a wonderful contrast that heightens the overall flavor profile. This deliberate interplay of tastes adds depth and complexity to foods, transforming them into sensory experiences.

The choice of cooking methods also plays a key role in making delectable meals. Techniques like roasting, grilling, and sautéing contribute diverse textures and savory overtones to ingredients. These procedures not only preserve the nutritional integrity of foods but also add a rich and tempting taste that enhances the overall enjoyment of the meal.

In the pursuit of maximum happiness, the composition of the plate becomes a canvas for culinary creativity. Incorporating a variety of textures—from the crispiness of roasted vegetables to the tenderness of well-cooked proteins—creates a dynamic and delightful dining experience. This diversity in textures lends an element of surprise and delight to each bite.

Mindful portioning helps to the overall enjoyment gained from meals. By intentionally serving adequate portions, folks can relish each bite without the unpleasantness of overeating. This practice coincides with the greater goal of establishing a balanced and healthful relationship with food, where pleasure and portion management coexist happily.

The combination of entire and nutrient-dense ingredients is vital to both flavor and satisfaction. Opting for fresh fruit, lean proteins, and whole grains not only boosts the nutritional content of meals but also lends a natural and nutritious taste. This intentional choice of ingredients guarantees that every bite contributes to both enjoyment and well-being.

Constructing meals for optimum flavor and enjoyment is an artful activity that demands a mindful blend of flavors, textures, and culinary methods. It is a chance to approach meal preparation with creativity and mindfulness, transforming each dining experience into a symphony of taste that nourishes both body and spirit.

Eating to best your diet plan

Setting off on a journey towards a healthy lifestyle frequently requires adopting a well-structured nutrition plan. Whether you're striving for weight control, higher energy levels, or overall well-being, learning how to eat to best support your diet plan is crucial to accomplishing your goals.

First and foremost, it's crucial to prioritize nutrient-dense foods. These are the powerhouse foods that carry a high concentration of vitamins, minerals, and other critical nutrients relative to their calorie intake. Fruits, vegetables, lean proteins, complete grains, and healthy fats should form the foundation of your meals. Not only do these foods provide the required building blocks for efficient physical processes, but they also contribute to a sensation of fullness and enjoyment.

Portion control plays a key part in aligning you're eating habits with your diet plan. Even the healthiest meals can lead to weight gain if consumed excessively. Understanding optimal portion sizes ensures that you're satisfying your nutritional needs without overloading your body with excessive calories. Consider integrating smaller, more frequent meals throughout the day to maintain energy levels and reduce overeating during larger meals.

Balancing macronutrients - proteins, lipids, and carbohydrates – is another key part of optimizing your food plan. Proteins are needed for muscle repair and maintenance, healthy fats provide continuous energy, and complex carbs supply a consistent flow of energy. Striking the appropriate balance between these macronutrients ensures that your body receives a full variety of nutrients for optimal functioning.

Meal timing can also influence the efficiency of your diet strategy. Eating at regular intervals helps balance blood sugar levels and minimizes strong hunger, reducing the likelihood of making unwise food choices. Consider spacing your meals and snacks equally throughout the day to maintain a continuous flow of energy.

Mindful eating is a discipline that compliments any diet plan. By being completely present throughout meals, you can create a stronger understanding of your body's hunger and fullness cues. This attention helps prevent overeating and produces a more joyful and gratifying meal experience. Avoid distractions like electronic devices and take the time to absorb the flavors, textures, and scents of your cuisine.

Hydration is often forgotten yet is a critical component of a healthy eating plan. Drinking a proper amount of water aids digestion, helps control appetite, and promotes general well-being. Consider making water your primary beverage and reduce the intake of sugary drinks and excessive caffeine.

Lastly, adaptation is crucial. While following a diet plan, be open to adjusting your strategy based on your body's responses and your evolving goals. Your nutritional demands may change over time, and a flexible approach allows you to make sustainable choices that match your long-term health objectives.

Eating to best support your diet plan comprises a smart blend of nutrient-dense meals, portion control, macronutrient balance, mindful eating practices, sufficient hydration, and a readiness to adjust. By integrating these ideas into your daily life, you may build a wholesome and sustainable eating regimen that increases your overall well-being.

Chapter 4

The Psychology of Indulgence

Understanding the psychology of indulgence uncovers the rich web of emotions, habits, and cognitive processes that drive our connection with decadent foods. It's a multidimensional examination of why we are driven to certain flavors, sensations, and experiences, and how our psychological landscape impacts our attitude to indulgence in a healthy and balanced manner.

At the foundation of indulgence lies the interplay of pleasure and reward within our brain's circuitry. Neurotransmitters such as dopamine, often associated with pleasure and reward, play a vital role. Indulging in meals that elicit a dopamine release provides a sensation of delight and fulfillment. However, noting the balance between occasional indulgence and general well-being is vital in navigating the psychology of these delightful experiences.

Emotional ties also weave into the psychology of indulgence. Food often intertwines with memories, comfort, and celebration, establishing a deep relationship between certain cuisines and emotional well-being. Recognizing these emotional ties encourages individuals to approach indulgence with awareness, separating emotional requirements from strictly physiological ones.

Cognitive elements, such as food cravings and the desire for diversity, contribute to the psychology of indulgence. Cravings may originate from a lack of specific nutrients or from conditioned responses to environmental signals. Understanding these indicators enables individuals to make informed choices, ensuring that indulgence matches with true needs rather than impulsive cravings.

The concept of mindful indulgence entails tasting each bite mindfully, allowing the sensory experience to emerge fully. Mindfulness allows folks to be present, experiencing the aromas and textures without falling into thoughtless overconsumption. This technique develops a better connection with rich foods, stressing quality over quantity.

Importantly, guilt and shame typically accompany gluttony, causing a negative psychological impact. It is crucial to build a mindset that views indulgence as a regular component of a balanced existence rather than a violation. By redefining the narrative around indulgence, individuals can enjoy these moments without the burden of unpleasant feelings.

The psychology of indulgence allows individuals to analyze their motivations, triggers, and responses to the enjoyment of eating. This awareness helps individuals to make informed choices, developing a relationship with indulgence that is both joyful and compatible with overall health and well-being. It's a voyage into the psyche, uncovering the nuances of our wants and impulses to build a balanced and fulfilling approach to decadent foods.

Breaking Free from Guilt and Food Shame

Breaking free from guilt and food shame is a transforming journey that entails altering the story surrounding our connection with food. It's an examination into understanding the inner intricacies and societal influences that often contribute to emotions of guilt and shame linked with food choices. By choosing a mindful and compassionate attitude, individuals can create a healthier connection with food and foster a good perspective.

Guilt and food shame typically come from cultural expectations, external judgments, or internalized views about what makes 'good' or 'poor' eating. It's vital to note that these concepts are sometimes arbitrary and can lead to a destructive cycle of restrictive eating followed by periods of overindulgence. The first step towards breaking free is to confront these ingrained assumptions and embrace a more flexible and balanced attitude toward food.

Understanding the concept of food neutrality can be a great aid in breaking free from guilt. This technique entails examining food without attaching moral significance. By reframing the attitude around some foods as neither fundamentally 'good' nor 'evil,' individuals can release the load of guilt associated with indulging. This shift allows for a more intuitive and aware approach to eating, where choices are chosen based on true appetites and nutritional needs.

Mindful eating habits serve a crucial role in reducing feelings of guilt and shame. By being present in the eating experience, savoring each mouthful, and paying attention to hunger and fullness signs, individuals can create a healthier connection with food. Mindfulness provides a non-judgmental awareness that dispels the negative feelings commonly linked with food choices.

Cultivating self-compassion is a critical element of breaking free from guilt. Recognizing that everyone has distinct nutritional demands and that occasional indulgence is a normal part of life helps cultivate a more forgiving and loving perspective. Instead of punishing oneself for perceived food violations, individuals should approach their choices with care and understanding.

Importantly, getting free from guilt entails letting go of the notion of 'perfect' eating. The pursuit of an optimal diet often leads to an unhealthy cycle of restriction and bingeing. Embracing imperfection and knowing that a balanced and diverse diet is the goal allows individuals to negotiate their relationship with food without the pressure of unreachable ideals.

Breaking free from guilt and eating shame is a liberating process that entails challenging conventional conventions, adopting mindful practices, and nurturing self-compassion. It's an opportunity to reinvent one's relationship with food, developing a positive and sustainable strategy that prioritizes total well-being and enjoyment.

Building a Positive Relationship with Food

Building a happy relationship with food is a transforming activity that requires modifying our thinking, actions, and emotions surrounding the act of eating. This journey is not about following tight diets or transient trends but about establishing a sustained and healthy connection with the food we consume.

Central to having a happy relationship with food is adopting the perspective of eating as fuel and nourishment. Recognizing that food is vital for sustaining life and promoting well-being shifts the focus from exterior judgments to internal demands. It allows consumers to appreciate the varied assortment of foods that contribute to general health without attributing moral worth to specific choices.

A vital factor in this path is increasing mindfulness during meals. Mindful eating means being fully present, relishing each bite, and paying attention to hunger and fullness indicators. This practice develops a non-judgmental awareness of the eating experience, building a deeper connection with the aromas, textures, and nutritional advantages of food. By embracing mindfulness, individuals can break free from the pattern of thoughtless eating and create a more intuitive approach to nourishment.

Embracing the concept of intuitive eating is crucial to having a happy connection with food. This technique encourages individuals to listen to their bodies, honor hunger and fullness, and respond to desires without guilt. Intuitive eating encourages a balanced and individualized approach to nutrition, encouraging individuals to make choices that accord with their physical and emotional well-being.

Positive self-talk has a crucial part in altering one's relationship with food. Instead of dwelling on restricted or negative thoughts, establishing a mentality of self-compassion and appreciation for the body's particular requirements can be revolutionary. Acknowledging that eating choices contribute to overall health without determining self-worth allows individuals to break free from the confines of cultural expectations.

Variety and moderation are pillars of a positive relationship with food. Embracing a vast range of meals ensures a broad spectrum of nutrients, while moderation allows for enjoyment without excess. By including a range of complete, nutrient-dense foods in meals, individuals can construct a balanced and fulfilling diet that supports both physical and mental well-being.

Creating a positive relationship with food is a holistic and ongoing process that incorporates mentality, actions, and self-compassion. It is an invitation to approach eating with joy, appreciation, and a clear knowledge of one's specific requirements. This journey leads to a sustained and rewarding connection with food, where nourishment becomes a source of pleasure, vitality, and overall well-being.

Treating Yourself: The Importance of Occasional Indulgence

Understanding the necessity of occasional indulgence is a cornerstone in establishing a balanced and sustainable attitude to eating. Contrary to conceptions of severe deprivation, occasional threats serve a key role in fostering both physical and mental well-being. Approaching excess with mindfulness and moderation can lead to a pleasant relationship with food, boosting the overall enjoyment of a healthy lifestyle.

Occasional indulgence is not synonymous with an abandonment of healthy practices; rather, it's an acknowledgment that a well-rounded approach to eating allows for flexibility and pleasure. Denying oneself the odd treat might lead to feelings of restriction, potentially sparking harmful eating patterns. Allowing leeway for indulgence minimizes the construction of rigid dietary norms, supporting a more natural and joyful attitude to eating.

The psychological benefits of occasional indulgence are remarkable. Treating yourself to a favorite dessert or comfort meal can bring a sense of joy and fulfillment, elevating spirits and adding to overall mental well-being. The act of indulgence, when done consciously, becomes a good and fulfilling experience, promoting a balanced perspective on food as a source of joy and nourishment.

From a physiological sense, occasional indulgence can prevent the pitfalls of continuous restriction. When individuals deny themselves the meals they crave, it may lead to an increased probability of overeating or bingeing later on. Allowing periodic rewards diminishes the temptation of forbidden foods and adds to a more sustainable and balanced relationship with eating.

The key to the importance of occasional indulgence lies in the concept of moderation. It's about enjoying treats in a controlled manner, appreciating each bite, and being conscious of portion proportions. This purposeful strategy allows consumers to receive pleasure from rich foods without compromising overall nutritional goals.

Moreover, occasional indulgence functions as a social and cultural connection. Sharing a special meal or enjoying a treat during festivities is a universal component of the human experience. It provides a sense of connection, allowing individuals to engage in collective delights without feeling alone or confined. This social component further highlights the good function that occasional indulgence can have in our lives.

Understanding the importance of occasional indulgence is about taking a balanced and mindful approach to eating. It is a knowledge that treats can be a source of joy, happiness, and connection when incorporated into a healthy lifestyle. By addressing indulgence with moderation and awareness, individuals can build a positive relationship with food that supports both their physical and emotional well-being.

Chapter 5

Culinary Creativity: Recipes for Indulgent Eating

Culinary creation is a palate-pleasing journey that transforms sumptuous eating into a joyful art form. Crafting dishes that highlight both flavor and nutrition is a skill that allows folks to experience the delights of indulgence while maintaining a healthful balance. By exploring unique culinary skills, one can increase the enjoyment of meals, turning them into pleasant and nourishing experiences.

A vital part of culinary innovation is the mindful selection of ingredients. Opting for full, nutrient-dense foods offers the foundation for delicious dishes that contribute to overall well-being. Incorporating a variety of colorful fruits, vegetables, lean proteins, and whole grains not only boosts the nutritional profile of recipes but also adds lively flavors and textures.

Experimenting with diverse cooking processes introduces an element of excitement to sumptuous cuisine. Grilling, roasting, or air-frying items can bring out unique flavors and textures, lending a wonderful touch to standard dishes. These strategies not only enhance the sensory experience of eating but also contribute to the overall enjoyment gained from lavish meals.

Balancing macronutrients is a critical factor in generating recipes for indulgent dining. Combining proteins, lipids, and carbohydrates in appropriate amounts ensures that meals are not only tasty but also satiating. This strategic balance provides a sensation of fullness, preventing the desire to overindulge, and creates a sense of satisfaction from each culinary creation.

Culinary inventiveness extends to the area of flavor combination. Exploring the harmonic blend of sweet, savory, and umami flavors adds depth and complexity to sumptuous meals. The skillful use of herbs, spices, and condiments can convert a simple dish into a culinary feast, illustrating that indulgence need not lose nutritional value.

Incorporating seasonal and local vegetables into dishes not only supports sustainability but also increases the freshness and flavor of meals. Seasonal ingredients provide a natural sweetness and vibrancy to dishes, allowing individuals to luxuriate in the richness of flavors while synchronizing with the ebb and flow of the culinary calendar.

Lastly, portion control remains a guiding guideline in the world of culinary inventiveness for indulgent dining.

Creating dishes with well-defined portion sizes encourages careful consumption and discourages overindulgence. This technique ensures that the pleasure received from each culinary creation is experienced in moderation, contributing to a balanced and healthful relationship with food.

gourmet innovation transforms luxurious dining into a gourmet adventure—one where flavors, textures, and nutrition combine in a pleasant symphony. By accepting this attitude, individuals can bask in the joy of indulgence without compromising their dedication to general health and well-being. It's a voyage into the art of savoring, where each recipe becomes a wonderful celebration of both taste and nourishment.

Flavourful Breakfasts to Kickstart Your Day

Setting off on a day with a breakfast that tantalizes the taste buds while feeding the body sets the foundation for a vibrant and invigorated morning. Crafting delectable breakfasts is an art that not only fulfills gourmet appetites but also delivers important nutrients to kickstart your day on a healthy note.

One wonderful and nutrient-packed alternative is the Greek yogurt parfait. Layering creamy Greek yogurt with a mix of fresh berries and a sprinkle of granola produces a morning symphony of textures and flavors. Rich in protein, probiotics, and antioxidants, this parfait not only pleases the mouth but also supports digestive health and maintains energy levels throughout the day.

For those seeking a savory start, an avocado and poached egg toast offer a delightful blend of tastes. The creamy avocado delivers healthful fats, while the poached egg adds a protein boost. Sprinkle with a sprinkle of chili flakes for an added kick, creating a breakfast that not only satisfies taste receptors but also contributes to fullness and prolonged attention.

Overnight oats present a time-saving yet delicious breakfast option. By soaking oats in your favorite milk or yogurt overnight and then topping them with fruits and nuts in the morning, you make a personalized and nutrient-dense meal. This meal is a source of complex carbs, fiber, and key vitamins, supporting a slow release of energy and keeping you nourished throughout the morning.

Exploring the world of smoothie bowls brings a rush of refreshing and colorful tastes to your breakfast routine. Blend a selection of fruits, greens, and a liquid base of your choosing, and top the smoothie with nuts, seeds, and oats for extra crunch. This colorful and nutrient-rich breakfast not only satisfies sweet cravings but also provides a variety of vitamins and minerals to enhance general well-being.

For those who prefer a warm start to the day, a veggie and quinoa breakfast skillet offers a delicious and robust option. Sautéing vegetables like bell peppers, spinach, and tomatoes with cooked quinoa provides a healthful and tasty dish. Top with a poached or fried egg for an extra protein boost, making it a wholesome and fulfilling breakfast meal.

Tasty breakfasts are a lovely way to enhance your mornings with energy and nourishment. These selections prove that breakfast can be both a gastronomic joy and a healthful choice. By introducing a range of nutrients and flavors into your morning routine, you set the tone for a day filled with vitality and happiness.

Satisfying Lunches that Fuel and Delight

Crafting fulfilling lunches that both fuel and delight is a culinary talent that transforms a midday meal into a moment of nourishment and fun. These alternatives go beyond ordinary sustenance, giving a symphony of flavors and nutrients to keep you energized and content throughout the day.

One healthful choice is the quinoa and vegetable Buddha bowl. Packed with a variety of bright veggies, and protein-rich quinoa, and topped with a tasty dressing, this bowl not only satisfies taste senses but also provides a balanced blend of vitamins, minerals, and vital amino acids. The broad array of nutrients enhances general well-being and sustains energy levels, making it a great choice for a fulfilling meal.

For those wanting a protein-packed choice, a grilled chicken salad with a vivid array of greens and toppings is both delicious and nutritious. The lean protein from the grilled chicken, mixed with an array of fresh veggies, makes a lunch that is not only satiating but also rich in vitamins and antioxidants. Tossing in a handful of nuts or seeds gives a wonderful crunch and an extra dose of healthy fats.

Embracing the world of plant-based possibilities, a chickpea and vegetable stir-fry gives a delicious combination of textures and flavors. Packed with protein and fiber, chickpeas add to a tasty and heart-healthy meal. Sautéing a selection of vibrant vegetables alongside the chickpeas provides a rush of vitamins and minerals, making a dinner that is both healthful and pleasant.

Another option that mixes both flavor and nutrition is the salmon and quinoa bowl. Grilled or baked salmon, rich in omega-3 fatty acids, mixes nicely with quinoa and a variety of veggies. This lunch pick not only delivers necessary nutrients for heart and brain health but also delights the taste buds with a flavorful and delicious combo.

For those who prefer the comfort of warm foods, a lentil and vegetable curry over brown rice gives a nourishing and savory lunch. Lentils give a plant-based protein supply while the assortment of spices in the curry provides depth and warmth to the dish. This selection not only satisfies the palette but also contributes to a well-rounded and healthful meal.

Satisfying lunches that fuel and thrill are a monument to the wonderful junction of flavor and nutrition. These selections indicate that a meal can be both a source of pleasure and a means of boosting general health. By

combining a range of nutrient-dense ingredients into your midday meals, you not only fulfill your appetite but also contribute to your well-being, producing a lunch experience that is both delicious and nourishing.

Decadent Dinners for Culinary Enjoyment

Creating extravagant dinners for gastronomic enjoyment is a fun exploration that transforms regular evenings into amazing dining experiences. These supper options not only satisfy the palette but also illustrate the harmonic interaction of flavors and nutrients, adding to both gastronomic delight and total well-being.

A decadent yet wholesome choice is the roasted veggie and quinoa-filled bell peppers. Packed with a medley of bright veggies, quinoa, and lean protein such as grilled chicken or tofu, this dish offers a symphony of textures and flavors. The nutritious density of the vegetables, along with the protein and fiber from quinoa, makes a supper that is both filling and nourishing.

Salmon en Papillote, a French culinary technique where the salmon is cooked in parchment paper, is a culinary marvel that lends elegance to the dinner table. Seasoned with herbs, lemon, and a drizzle of olive oil, this dish not only maintains the delicate aromas of the salmon but also offers a high supply of omega-3 fatty acids, contributing to heart and brain health.

For those with a fondness for plant-based treats, a wild mushroom risotto is a savory and decadent alternative. Arborio rice cooked to creamy perfection with a variety of wild mushrooms, a splash of white wine, and vegetable broth creates a dish that exemplifies the art of culinary simplicity and richness. The earthy flavors of mushrooms, paired with the creaminess of the risotto, create for a dinner that is both comforting and refined.

An herb-infused grilled lamb chops choice offers a touch of refinement to the dinner table. Marinated in a blend of fresh herbs, garlic, and olive oil, the lamb chops are grilled to perfection, providing a succulent and savory main dish. This supper choice not only pleases the senses but also delivers a quality supply of protein and necessary nutrients.

Exploring the world of plant-based alternatives, lentil, and sweet potato curry gives a rush of exotic aromas and heartiness. Lentils, rich in protein and fiber, mixed with the sweetness of sweet potatoes and a blend of aromatic spices, produce a dish that is not only tasty but also a nutritious powerhouse. The harmonic balance of ingredients makes this dinner a delightful adventure into plant-based culinary ingenuity.

Decadent dinners for culinary enjoyment prove that excess and health can coexist on the dinner plate. These alternatives represent the artistry of designing meals that thrill the taste buds while supplying critical nutrients for overall well-being. By introducing a varied assortment of products and cooking techniques into your nightly meals, you elevate the dining experience, turning it into a celebration of both flavor and nourishment.

Irresistible Snacks and Desserts

Indulging in alluring snacks and desserts can be a delightful experience when undertaken with a mindful and healthful viewpoint. These scrumptious solutions not only satisfy sweet cravings but also highlight that flavorful snacks may coincide with a balanced and healthful lifestyle.

For a guilt-free snack, a handful of mixed nuts is a great choice. Rich in healthy fats, protein, and a variety of critical components, nuts give a delicious crunch while boosting satiety. Whether almonds, walnuts, or cashews, this snack offers a combination of heart-healthy advantages with a natural sweetness that makes it both delicious and nutritious.

When it comes to sweets, choosing for a fruit-based dish like a berry parfait strikes a nice mix between sweetness and healthfulness. Layering fresh berries with Greek yogurt and a drizzle of honey or a sprinkling of oats creates a dessert that is not only visually pleasing but also rich in antioxidants, probiotics, and vitamins. This delight fulfills the sweet desire while giving a refreshing and healthful experience.

Dark chocolate-dipped strawberries give a tasty yet wholesome dessert alternative. Dark chocolate, with its antioxidant characteristics, pairs nicely with the natural sweetness of strawberries. The combination not only satisfies appetites for a rich treat but also benefits cardiovascular health and delivers a dose of important minerals.

For those wanting a delicious snack with a healthier twist, oven-baked sweet potato fries are a delightful choice. Slice sweet potatoes into fries, toss them in olive oil and a sprinkle of spices, then bake until crispy. This snack not only satisfies the craving for a savory delight but also gives a nutrient-dense alternative to regular potato fries, delivering a boost of vitamins and fiber.

Indulging in a coconut chia pudding as a dessert is a great way to merge flavor with nutrition. Combining coconut milk, chia seeds, and a dash of natural sweetness creates a creamy and delightful pudding. This dessert not only satiates sweet cravings but also gives a dose of healthy fats, fiber, and plant-based proteins, making it a well-rounded and pleasurable choice.

Irresistible snacks and sweets need not be linked with excess at the expense of health. These selections prove that cautious decisions may still be immensely fun. By combining a range of nutrient-dense ingredients into your snacks and sweets, you not only indulge your taste buds but also contribute to your general well-being, providing a pleasurable and beneficial experience that delights both the palate and body.

Chapter 6

Dining Out Without Derailing Your Goals

An individual's ability to navigate restaurant menus while sticking to their health and wellness goals is a skill that enables them to enjoy dining out without compromising their goals. Through the adoption of a conscious and informed attitude, you will be able to enjoy the experience of dining out while simultaneously making decisions that are in line with your health goals.

In order to get started with your dining trip, you need to first carefully examine the menu. Look for dishes that highlight lean proteins, nutritious grains, and an abundance of vegetables. Opting for grilled or roasted choices rather than fried can drastically reduce the total calorie and fat load of your meal.

It is recommended that you start with a salad or a soup that is based on broth when it comes to selecting an appetizer. The consumption of these options not only increases the amount of vegetables you consume, but they also make you feel fuller, which makes it easier for you to avoid overindulging in the main course. It is important to exercise caution when it comes to dressings and choose vinaigrettes or ask for them on the side in order to control the amount.

When it comes to a dining experience that is focused on health, the most important thing is to have main dishes that include a wide range of colorful vegetables and lean proteins. Fish that has been grilled, lean cuts of meat, or plant-based proteins such as tofu are all potential fantastic options. If you ask for sauces and dressings to be served on the side, you will have the ability to regulate the amount that you take, which will allow you to enjoy the flavors without going overboard.

When it is practicable, you should embrace the art of substitution. Swap out high-calorie sides like fries for steamed veggies, or opt for brown rice instead of white. Many restaurants are agreeable to such requests, contributing to a healthier and more balanced dinner.

Mindful portion control is key. Consider splitting dishes or packaging up half of your meal at the beginning. This strategy not only minimizes overeating but also provides a pleasant opportunity to taste the food on another day.

When it comes to beverages, pick water or herbal teas over sugary sodas or calorie-laden cocktails. Staying hydrated with water promotes digestion and ensures you're not accidentally taking more calories through beverages.

Lastly, don't shy away from dessert. Sharing a dessert or picking options like fresh fruit, sorbet, or a modest dish of a lighter treat allows you to enjoy a sweet finale without derailing your health goals.

Dining out can be an enjoyable and health-conscious experience when handled with care. By making careful decisions and maintaining balance, you may savor the pleasures of restaurant cuisine while keeping connected with your wellness goals. It's a technique that transforms dining out into a celebration of both taste and health, proving that the enjoyment of food need not compromise your dedication to well-being.

Navigating Restaurant Menus for Indulgent Choices

When presented with a restaurant menu, the quest for indulgent choices need not be a compromising venture on your health and fitness journey. A careful approach to navigating menus helps you to delight in the pleasures of dining out while still choosing choices that match your health goals.

Start your culinary journey by examining the menu for terms that signify better preparation methods. Look for phrases like grilled, roasted, or steamed, which frequently indicate a milder cooking style. Dishes prepared utilizing these methods tend to be lower in added fats and calories, offering a base for indulgence without excessive compromise.

Consider beginning your dining experience with a bright and nutrient-packed salad. Opt for meals that offer a range of colorful vegetables, lean proteins, and a variety of textures. This not only serves as a great appetizer but also helps with your daily intake of vitamins and minerals.

When it comes to main meals, don't shy away from protein-rich selections. Grilled fish, lean cuts of meat, or plant-based proteins can be decadent options that correspond with your dietary goals. Be cautious of portion sizes and relish each bite, enabling yourself to enjoy the tastes without the desire for excess.

Embrace the variety of vegetable sides. Restaurants often provide a menu of side dishes utilizing seasonal vegetables. These can be a tasty and beneficial addition to your sumptuous meal, providing necessary nutrients and fiber while enriching the whole eating experience.

Be cautious with thick sauces and condiments. Opt for foods with milder, broth-based sauces, or ask for dressings on the side. This strategy allows you to regulate the number of additional fats and calories while still experiencing the flavors of the food.

If you find yourself enticed by dessert, try sharing it with your dining mates. In this manner, you can satisfy your sweet desire without overindulging. Alternatively, investigate fruit-based sweets or options with lighter ingredients to create a balance between enjoyment and health.

Navigating restaurant menus for decadent selections is a skill that blends the fun of dining out with a commitment to wellness. By making informed and intentional choices, you can transform your restaurant experience into a celebration of both gourmet delight and health-conscious choices. It's a voyage that illustrates that the pursuit of pleasure need not compromise your dedication to a good and balanced life.

Socializing and Celebrating with Smart Food Choices

Socializing and celebrating often involve food, and making sensible choices during these events can increase your well-being without reducing the excitement of the moment. By adopting an informed and balanced approach, you may navigate gatherings and festivities while making decisions that match your health goals.

When attending social events, start by assessing the offerings and making conscious selections. Opt for a plate that offers a mix of colorful veggies, lean proteins, and nutritious grains. This not only maintains a balance of nutrients but also helps you to experience the varied flavors supplied.

Consider portion control as a major tactic. While enjoying the assortment of dishes provided, be cautious of your portions. Take the time to savor each bite, appreciating the textures and flavors. This method not only supports your health goals but also helps you to completely enjoy the culinary experience.

Choose prudently when it comes to beverages. Opt for water, herbal teas, or sparkling water with a splash of citrus instead of sugary sodas or excessive amounts of alcohol. Staying hydrated not only benefits general health but also aids in reducing calorie intake.

When faced with dessert selections, explore lighter choices or share with others. Fresh fruit, a small portion of a less decadent delicacy, or sharing a dessert allows you to join in the celebration component without overindulging in sweets.

Engage in the social side of the gathering rather than focusing simply on the food. Conversations, laughter, and the enjoyment of the company contribute substantially to the whole experience. By concentrating on the social side, you might discover joy beyond only the culinary delights.

Consider contributing to the celebration by bringing a healthier cuisine. Whether it's a vibrant salad, a vegetable-based starter, or a fruit plate, giving nutritional options guarantees there's something healthy for everyone to enjoy.

Practice awareness during celebrations. Be alert to your body's hunger and fullness cues, and know when you've eaten enough. This awareness allows you to make choices that are in harmony with your body's requirements.

Interacting and celebrating with smart food choices is an art that combines the joy of shared times with a commitment to well-being. By taking a mindful approach, you may navigate parties with confidence, selecting choices that honor both your health goals and the festive spirit of the occasion. It's a technique that sweetens the experience of socializing, making each celebration a pleasurable and healthy affair.

Tips for Enjoyable and Guilt-Free Eating at Events

Approaching events and gatherings with an emphasis on pleasurable and guilt-free eating takes a blend of awareness, informed decisions, and a healthy relationship with food. By implementing these guidelines, you can savor the social side of events while honoring your well-being.

Begin by establishing a balanced mindset. Approach events to enjoy both the food and the company. Acknowledge that occasional indulgence is a natural part of life, and it need not be accompanied by guilt. Embrace that a single event does not define your overall eating habits.

Survey the offerings with a careful eye. Take a minute to analyze the meal alternatives before digging in. Choose a well-rounded plate that includes a variety of veggies, lean proteins, and nutritious grains. This ensures a range of nutrients and flavors while contributing to a sense of satiety.

Practice mindful eating. Engage your senses by savoring each bite, and appreciating the textures and tastes. Eating slowly permits your body to sense fullness, limiting overindulgence. Conversations and interactions throughout the occasion might be just as enjoyable as the food itself.

Opt for moderation in your decisions. While it's tempting to sample everything, consider smaller servings of rich meals. This way, you can enjoy the flavors without feeling overwhelmed or jeopardizing your health goals. Be aware of portion sizes, allowing oneself to savor the event without excess.

Stay hydrated throughout the event. Water not only promotes digestion but also helps moderate hunger. Sipping water between bites might enhance the entire experience and contribute to a feeling of fullness.

Be selective with your alcohol consumption. If you use to drink, do so in moderation way. Alcoholic beverages can offer significant calories, and excess intake may lead to less conscious eating. Alternating alcoholic drinks with water can assist in regulating both calorie intake and hydration.

Contribute healthier options to the celebration. If appropriate, volunteer to bring food that corresponds with your health goals. This ensures you have a healthy option available, plus it also presents a nice gesture to those who may have similar tastes.

Lastly, let go of any guilt correlated with enjoying rare pleasures. Remember that guilt-free eating is not about restriction but rather about balance and thoughtful decisions.

Combining these principles allows you to savor events with a sense of joy, appreciation, and commitment to your general well-being.

Chapter 7

Fitness and Fun: Balancing Activity with Indulgence

Balancing indulgence with physical activity is a dynamic approach to wellness that not only develops a healthy lifestyle but also injects an element of delight into workout regimens. Striking this balance is vital for general well-being, as it allows you to enjoy the pleasures of indulgence while supporting your body with the benefits of exercise.

Start by rethinking your perspective on exercise. Instead of considering it only as a tool to burn calories, consider it an opportunity to engage in things that provide joy and contentment. Whether it's a dance class, a nature trip, or a bike ride, choosing activities you actually enjoy transforms exercise into a pleasurable experience.

Incorporate variation into your fitness program. Engaging in numerous activities not only eliminates boredom but also targets different muscle areas, adding to overall physical wellness. Whether it's cardio, weight training, or flexibility exercises, a well-rounded routine provides overall fitness.

Align your fitness program with your indulgent moments. If you anticipate a special dinner or event, arrange your exercise program accordingly. This proactive approach not only enables indulgence but also develops a healthy link between food and exercise, emphasizing balance rather than restriction.

Explore group activities or classes. Participating in group exercise endeavors provides an element of enjoyment and accountability. Whether it's a group workout class, team sports, or simply exercising with a friend, the communal aspect can convert physical activity into a shared, pleasurable experience.

Consider introducing playful elements into your training program. Activities like recreational sports, dance, or even playful workouts can impart a sense of delight, making exercise feel less like a chore and more like a source of pleasure.

Celebrate victories, both big and small. Recognizing success in your fitness journey, whether it's greater stamina, strength, or flexibility, maintains a favorable association with physical activity. Regular acknowledgment of your efforts creates a mindset that enjoys the rewards of a healthy, active lifestyle.

Be adaptive with your fitness routine. Life is energetic, and so should be your style to exercise. If a regular gym workout doesn't appeal to you, explore alternatives like outdoor activities, home workouts, or even trying new sports. This versatility means that fitness stays a source of delight rather than a rigid requirement.

Balancing action with pleasure is about building a sustainable and pleasurable approach to both fitness and wellness. By finding enjoyment in physical activity and embracing the multiplicity of exercise possibilities, you develop a harmonious lifestyle that celebrates the joy of movement while providing room for indulgence moments. This balanced approach not only adds to physical health but also increases your total sense of well-being.

The Role of Exercise in a Balanced Lifestyle

Exercise, far beyond being a simple physical activity, is a keystone of a healthy lifestyle that extends its effect into different areas of well-being. Its purpose is not confined to sculpting the body; rather, it intertwines with mental, emotional, and even social components, leading to a comprehensive sense of health and vitality.

At its foundation, exercise is a potent instrument for physical fitness. Engaging in regular physical activity boosts cardiovascular health, develops muscles, and supports the maintenance of a healthy body weight. It becomes a dynamic means of bolstering the body's structural base and developing resilience against numerous health challenges.

Yet the advantages of exercise extend well beyond the physical sphere. There is an intrinsic relationship between physical activity and mental well-being. Regular exercise has been connected to reduced stress, anxiety, and depression. The release of endorphins, sometimes referred to as "feel-good" hormones, during physical activity contributes to an improved mood and an enhanced sense of general mental wellness.

Moreover, exercise is a catalyst for cognitive function. It has been connected with higher cognitive capacities, including greater memory and attention span. The act of exercising the body stimulates the brain, generating an interplay between physical and mental fitness that highlights the necessity of a well-rounded approach to health.

In the framework of a healthy lifestyle, exercise becomes a tool for stress management. Amidst the demands of modern life, physical activity serves as a natural stress reliever, allowing a sanctuary for people to decompress, clear their minds, and achieve equilibrium. It becomes a meditative exercise, developing a mindful connection between the body and the present moment.

Beyond its benefits, exercise may be a community undertaking, adding to a sense of social well-being. Group activities, team sports, or gym classes give opportunities for social interaction, building a sense of camaraderie and connection. The common experience of achieving fitness objectives can deepen connections and form a supportive community.

The significance of exercise in a healthy lifestyle is diverse. It is a fundamental factor in the pursuit of physical health, mental well-being, and emotional balance. It serves as a tool for stress relief, cognitive enhancement, and a means to create social connections. By embracing exercise as an intrinsic part of daily life, individuals can create a harmonious and holistic approach to their overall well-being, sweetening the journey towards a healthier and more happy life.

Finding Activities, You Enjoy

Setting off on a fitness path is a personal exploration that can be substantially sweetened by finding things that bring joy and fulfillment. The key to keeping a long-term commitment to exercise rests in discovering forms of physical activity that resonate with your preferences and lifestyle, changing fitness from a chore into a gratifying and delightful experience.

Consider this journey as an opportunity to try diverse activities. From classic workouts like jogging or weightlifting to more offbeat options like dancing, hiking, or martial arts, the number of possibilities is extensive. Sampling diverse activities allows you to identify those that resonate with your interests, making the pursuit of fitness a fascinating and ever-evolving experience.

Reflect on prior experiences that brought joy and movement into your life. Whether it's childhood sports, recreational interests, or even playful activities, these examples offer pointers about activities that correspond with your inclinations. Revisiting the past can revive a sense of delight, making exercise a nostalgic and joyful undertaking.

Explore group or community activities. Joining fitness programs, group sports, or workout groups offers a social element that can considerably boost the enjoyment of exercise. The companionship and shared experiences create a supportive environment, turning physical activity into a social and uplifting affair.

Consider the surroundings. The natural world offers a plethora of options for physical activity, from hiking paths to coastal runs. Exploring outdoor activities not only links you with nature but also provides an element of novelty and fun to your workout program.

Tailor your activities to your mood and energy levels. Some days may call for high-intensity workouts, while others may be better suited to calmer pursuits like yoga or cycling. Understanding your body's signs and changing your routine accordingly ensures that exercise remains a flexible and pleasurable part of your everyday life.

Integrate variation into your routine. Monotony can lead to boredom and apathy. By adding diverse activities throughout the week, you keep your routine fresh and entertaining. This variation not only minimizes burnout but also exposes you to a range of physical benefits.

Finding activities, you enjoy is about enjoying movement as a source of enjoyment and well-being. By matching exercise with your hobbies, tastes, and social ties, you infuse your fitness journey with a feeling of joy. This technique converts physical activity from a mere responsibility into a joyful and lasting practice, sweetening the way toward a healthier and more fulfilling existence

Creating a Sustainable Exercise Routine

Creating a sustainable exercise regimen is analogous to constructing a blueprint for long-term well-being, presenting a path that is both practical and enjoyable. This road towards fitness is not a momentary commitment but rather a continual, sustained practice that harmonizes with your lifestyle, ensuring enduring health advantages.

Begin by creating reasonable and achievable goals. These objectives should coincide with your fitness aspirations, whether they involve weight control, improved cardiovascular health, or enhanced overall well-being. Realistic goals create a tangible framework, allowing you to monitor progress and celebrate victories, establishing a positive feedback loop.

Integrate variation into your routine. Monotony can be a substantial impediment to long-term adherence. By incorporating varied activities—such as cardio, strength training, flexibility exercises, and leisure sports—your regimen remains dynamic and entertaining. This variation not only eliminates boredom but also promotes a well-rounded approach to fitness, emphasizing different facets of physical health.

Consider the notion of progressive growth. While enthusiasm may encourage you to embrace difficult workouts from the outset, a steady increase in intensity and length helps your body to adapt. This method lowers the chance of burnout or injury, making the journey towards fitness a sustainable and injury-free activity.

Prioritize consistency above intensity. Sustainable exercise is not about pushing your body to its limits every day but rather keeping a consistent habit. Consistency supports habit building, transforming physical activity into a vital part of your everyday life. Aim for a balance that meets your schedule, making exercise a realistic and feasible commitment.

Incorporate flexibility into your regimen. Life is lively, and so should be your approach to exercise. Recognize that there will be days when your schedule is tight or when your body needs rest. A flexible program allows you to adjust so that fitness stays a source of enjoyment rather than a rigid responsibility.

Embrace the concept of active living. Physical activity extends beyond traditional workout routines. Incorporate movement into your daily life, whether it's using the stairs, going for a stroll during breaks, or engaging in active hobbies. This holistic approach incorporates fitness effortlessly into your lifestyle, making it more sustainable in the long run.

Make your routine joyful. Identify activities that provide delight and fulfillment. Whether it's dancing, hiking, or playing a sport, finding pleasure in your chosen hobbies transforms fitness from a chore into a source of delight. Enjoyment not only sweetens the journey but also reinforces a favorable relationship with fitness.

By weaving these ideas into the fabric of your training program, you build a sustainable and durable approach to fitness. It is not a transitory commitment but a lifelong practice that harmonizes with your lifestyle, guaranteeing that the journey towards well-being is not only healthful but also delightful.

Chapter 8

Overcoming Common Challenges

Embarking on a journey toward a better lifestyle frequently comes with its share of hurdles. Recognizing and overcoming these typical hurdles is an important component of sustaining a healthy and sustainable attitude to well-being.

One recurrent difficulty is the hurdle of time limits. Modern life can be stressful, leaving limited space for concentrated workout sessions. To overcome this, consider combining shorter, high-intensity workouts into your regimen or splitting lengthier sessions into manageable portions throughout the day. Efficient and effective workouts can fit effortlessly into busy schedules.

Another stumbling hurdle is the all-or-nothing approach. Some people feel disappointed if they miss a workout or indulge in an occasional pleasure. It's crucial to remember that consistency over time matters more than occasional setbacks. Adopting a flexible mindset, where occasional deviations are regarded as part of a healthy life, minimizes feelings of guilt and fosters a healthier relationship with exercise and nutrition.

Finding motivation can be a constant issue. To solve this, develop realistic and meaningful goals that resonate with your values. Whether it's increasing energy levels, managing stress, or attaining specific fitness milestones, having a clear sense of purpose may fuel motivation. Additionally, consider combining activities you enjoy, converting fitness from a chore into a source of enjoyment.

Injuries and physical restrictions can be substantial hurdles on the path to well-being. It's vital to listen to your body, alter activities as needed, and consult with healthcare specialists or fitness experts to build a safe and individualized plan. Approaching exercise with mindfulness and adapting to your body's needs guarantees a sustained and injury-free journey.

Nutritional issues typically accompany fitness ambitions. Overcoming the appeal of unhealthy snacks or limiting portion sizes demands a balanced and attentive approach. Aim for a broad and nutrient-rich diet, emphasizing whole foods. Developing a balanced relationship with food, where indulgences are enjoyed in moderation, develops a sustainable and guilt-free nutritional lifestyle.

Lastly, social and environmental factors can influence your health journey. Peer pressure, societal expectations, or a lack of accessible exercise resources may offer obstacles. Building a supporting network, seeking like-minded individuals, and exploring creative solutions—such as at-home workouts or outdoor activities—help overcome external constraints and cultivate a good and encouraging environment.

Acknowledging and tackling these obstacles as vital components of the wellness journey enables a more resilient and sustainable approach to healthy living. By negotiating these typical difficulties with mindfulness, adaptability, and a positive perspective, you not only sweeten the route but also establish a foundation for long-term well-being and contentment.

Dealing with Emotional Eating

Balancing emotional eating is a delicate component of well-being that involves both self-awareness and compassionate understanding. Emotions can sometimes become interwoven with our connection with food, leading to a cycle of comfort-seeking through eating. Developing skills to cope with emotional eating is vital for maintaining a healthy and balanced attitude to nutrition.

Firstly, it's necessary to identify the reasons for emotional eating. Pay attention to the emotions, situations, or anxieties that drive the impulse to indulge in comfort foods. Understanding these triggers allows you to address the fundamental cause of emotional eating, enabling more effective coping techniques.

Mindfulness appears as a powerful weapon in the struggle against emotional eating. Cultivating awareness of your thoughts, emotions, and physical sensations during eating helps break the reflexive response to emotional cues. By enjoying each bite, you enrich the sensory experience of eating and build a more intentional and mindful relationship with food.

Developing alternative coping methods is crucial for channeling emotional impulses away from eating. Engaging in activities such as meditation, deep breathing exercises, or physical activities provides better outlets for managing stress and emotions. Establishing a toolkit of alternate tactics helps you respond to emotional situations without resorting to food as the default coping mechanism.

Creating a supportive workplace is equally vital. Surround yourself with persons who understand and respect your wellness goals. Communicate with friends or family about your adventure, and seek their encouragement. Having a solid support system can help you stay accountable and reward beneficial actions.

Distinguishing between physical hunger and emotional hunger is a critical skill in conquering emotional eating. True physical hunger develops gradually and can be met with a range of nutrient-rich foods. Emotional hunger, on the other hand, tends to want specific comfort foods. By tuning into your body's cues, you may make more informed choices about when and what to consume.

Building a positive relationship with food requires reducing the stigma frequently linked with emotional eating. Take that occasional emotional eating is a normal part of life. Instead of carrying shame, focus on learning from these events and using them as chances for growth and self-discovery.

Dealing with emotional eating involves a holistic strategy that incorporates self-awareness, mindfulness, and compassionate understanding. By embracing healthy coping techniques, cultivating a happy atmosphere, and changing your connection with food, you may sweeten the road toward a balanced and emotionally intelligent approach to nutrition.

Handling Plateaus and Setbacks

Setting out on a path toward a healthy lifestyle is a praiseworthy undertaking, but it's not uncommon to meet plateaus and setbacks along the road. These situations, albeit tough, present important possibilities for growth and resilience. Let's explore effective ways of addressing plateaus and failures with grace and determination.

Firstly, it's crucial to understand that plateaus are a natural part of any wellness journey. Whether in exercise or nutrition, your body may reach a point where progress seems to stagnate. Instead of perceiving plateaus as hurdles, consider them as indications for future modifications. Reassess your workout program, modify your food choices, or explore new forms of exercise to promote fresh development.

Setbacks, on the other hand, can be upsetting but are not symptomatic of failure. Life is unpredictable, and numerous factors—such as stress, illness, or unexpected events—can disturb your schedule. Instead of concentrating on setbacks, regard them as momentary detours. Adopt a resilient mindset that accepts failure, learns from it, and recalibrates your strategy moving ahead.

Maintaining a positive outlook during plateaus and failures is key. Cultivate a mindset that focuses on the long journey rather than fixating on short-term volatility. Celebrate the progress you've achieved, the lessons gained, and the dedication to long-term well-being. This positive mindset can act as a tremendous motivator to overcome problems.

Plateaus typically highlight the need for variety in your training regimen. Introduce new exercises, switch up your workout intensity, or explore different forms of physical activity. This not only keeps things interesting but also challenges your body in novel ways, breaking through performance plateaus.

In nutrition, plateaus may emerge from monotony or an imbalance in nutritional consumption. Evaluate your nutritional choices, ensuring a wide and nutrient-rich assortment of foods. Incorporating a diverse array of fruits, vegetables, lean proteins, and whole grains delivers critical nutrients and enhances general well-being.

During setbacks, maintaining constancy in your efforts is vital. Rather than succumbing to discouragement, use failures as chances to reassess your goals, adapt your techniques, and enhance your dedication. Resilience in the face of setbacks is a hallmark of a sustainable and successful wellness journey.

Finally, seek support during hard circumstances. Share your experiences with friends, family, or a fitness community. Surrounding oneself with support and understanding promotes a sense of camaraderie and helps you stay motivated through plateaus and disappointments.

Navigating plateaus and setbacks is a vital aspect of any health and fitness journey. By tackling these moments with adaptability, a positive outlook, and a commitment to long-term well-being, you not only overcome problems but also sweeten the whole experience of obtaining a healthier and happier living.

Staying Motivated for Long-Term Success

Sustaining motivation over the long term is a tough yet necessary component of any journey toward enduring health and wellness. While initial enthusiasm might drive beneficial changes, the key comes in building habits and mindsets that last the test of time. Here, we discuss practical techniques to keep the spark of inspiration burning for sustainable achievement.

Firstly, creating realistic and individualized goals is crucial. Rather than fixating on rapid, dramatic changes, develop reasonable objectives that match your circumstances. Break down major objectives into smaller, achievable milestones, providing a roadmap that allows for consistent development and lowers the chance of burnout.

A dynamic and diverse routine can substantially contribute to prolonged motivation. In both fitness and diet, monotony may be a motivation killer. Incorporate diverse workouts, explore new dishes, and promote alternative forms of physical activity. This not only keeps things interesting but also challenges your body and mind, preventing the emergence of boredom or stagnation.

Tracking progress is a highly motivational tool. Regularly monitor your achievements, whether it's increases in exercise levels, nutritional milestones, or changes in overall well-being. Tangible evidence of progress acts as a reminder of how far you've gone, confirming your dedication and driving continued work.

Cultivating a good perspective is crucial in retaining motivation. Focus on the benefits of a healthy lifestyle beyond physical appearance, such as greater energy, improved mood, and enhanced general well-being. By shifting the emphasis from outward validation to internal satisfaction, you develop a durable basis for long-term success.

Incorporating elements of joy into your wellness journey adds a lovely layer to the process. Find activities you enjoy, be it a favorite sport, a dance class, or a leisurely nature walk. Infusing joy into your routine transforms travel from a perceived responsibility into a source of pure satisfaction.

Social support plays a critical part in sustaining motivation. Surround yourself with like-minded others, whether through fitness programs, online communities, or workout pals. Sharing experiences, struggles, and achievements fosters a sense of camaraderie, reinforcing your commitment to health and fitness.

It's vital to realize that setbacks are a natural part of any journey. Rather than perceiving them as insurmountable challenges, perceive them as excellent learning opportunities. Cultivating resilience in the face of adversity is a testimonial to your passion and perseverance for long-term success.

Being motivated for long-term success is about finding a balance between discipline and flexibility. Embrace the path as a continuous exploration of self-improvement, where each day brings a chance to make choices that correspond with your wellness goals. By developing a positive outlook, praising progress, and infusing joy into your routine, you sweeten the route to enduring health and fulfillment.

Chapter 9

Embracing the Journey

A fundamental commitment to oneself, an investment in well-being that goes beyond simple physical transformation, is required in order to get started on the journey toward a life that is healthier and more satisfying. Embracing a comprehensive journey that nourishes both the body and the mind is not simply about losing weight or finding a short-term solution; rather, it is about embracing a holistic journey.

The journey that you are about to begin is a celebration of self-discovery, and each step is an opportunity to investigate the various layers of your potential. You should not consider the road that lies ahead to be a difficult obstacle; rather, you should consider it to be a thrilling exploration of your talents, an adventure in which you are both the navigator and the destination.

The journey is not about imposing strict regulations or harsh measures; rather, it is about developing a way of life that is congruent with your unique traits and characteristics. This is an invitation to explore the joy that can be found in exercise, the pleasure that can be found in nourishing your body with nutrients that are good for you, and the fulfillment that can be obtained from building a positive relationship with yourself. The journey that you are on is one that thrives on simplicity, finding happiness in the most fundamental yet profound acts of self-care.

During this journey, obstacles are not obstacles; rather, they are gentle nudges to reevaluate and adapt one's course of action. In other words, it is about accepting the ups and downs of life and acknowledging that every moment, regardless of whether it is a triumph or a challenge, adds to the overall depth of your experience. The journey that we are on places a higher emphasis on progress than perfection, recognizing that the road to happiness is not a straight line but rather a tapestry that is weaved with a variety of different threads of effort and perseverance.

Moreover, this excursion is a testimonial to the power of awareness. It encourages you to taste each bite, relish every step, and be present on the trip rather than fixating on the destination. The beauty is not only in the end objective but also in the daily rituals and habits that create your route.

As you traverse this trip, know that you are not alone. Connect with a community of fellow travelers, exchanging thoughts, problems, and achievements. The collaborative strength and support establish an environment where growth develops, making the expedition all the more enriching.

Embrace this adventure with open arms, allowing it to evolve naturally and truthfully. Cherish the moments of self-discovery, relish the flavor of wholesome foods, and delight in the thrill of movement. This is not only a quest for physical well-being; it is an endeavor to develop a harmonious connection with yourself, to sweeten the chapters of your life with the richness of health and fulfillment.

Celebrating Small Victories

In the pursuit of a healthier and more balanced life, it's vital to celebrate small wins along the way. These moments, seemingly little, are the building blocks of sustainable change and should be valued for the enormous impact they have on your well-being.

Consider every nutritious meal, every thoughtful bite, and every step taken towards an active lifestyle as an accomplishment worth celebrating. By acknowledging these modest accomplishments, you establish a positive reinforcement loop, developing a mindset that values progress over perfection.

Small successes often act as signposts on your wellness path, suggesting that you are headed in the right way. Whether it's choosing a nutritious snack over a sugary temptation or finishing a workout, each victory is a tribute to your commitment to self-improvement.

Moreover, admiring such occurrences cultivates a sense of gratitude for your body and the work done in its care. Recognizing the significance of tiny triumphs instills a sense of accomplishment, pushing you to persist in the face of obstacles.

These achievements transcend the physical realm, influencing your mental and emotional well-being. They encourage your ability to make positive choices and promote the notion that sustainable transformation is built upon a foundation of persistent, focused acts.

While the great destination of maximum health may be the ultimate aim, the route is peppered with these enjoyable milestones. Embrace them with gusto, realizing that they add greatly to the grand tapestry of your general well-being.

In celebrating little triumphs, you not only recognize your progress but also build resilience against setbacks. It creates a continual loop of positive reinforcement, where one achievement fuels the momentum for the next, producing a sustainable and rewarding journey towards a healthier, happier you.

So, take a moment to savor these accomplishments. Whether it's fighting the impulse to indulge in unhealthy behaviors or just choosing to prioritize self-care, each small triumph is a monument to your dedication and a crucial thread in the fabric of your well-lived existence.

Shifting from Dieting to Sustainable Lifestyle Choices

Embarking on a journey toward a healthier, more balanced lifestyle is a profound shift—one that transcends the transient nature of diets and embraces the sustainable tapestry of mindful choices. In our quest for well-being, it's essential to recognize the limitations of traditional dieting approaches and instead focus on cultivating sustainable lifestyle habits that stand the test of time.

Dieting often implies temporary restrictions and rigid rules that can be both physically and mentally taxing. It's a short-term solution to a long-term goal, often leaving individuals feeling trapped in a cycle of deprivation and indulgence. The key lies in transitioning from this restrictive mindset to a sustainable lifestyle that is both nourishing and enjoyable.

The shift from dieting to sustainable lifestyle choices is rooted in the understanding that health is not a destination but a continuous journey. It involves making choices that align with your long-term well-being rather than succumbing to the allure of quick fixes. Instead of fixating on short-term goals, focus on building habits that contribute to a sustainable, health-focused lifestyle.

Consider adopting a holistic approach that encompasses nutrition, exercise, and mental well-being. Rather than looking food as the enemy, embrace it as a source of nourishment and pleasure. Choose nutrient-dense, whole foods that not only fuel your body but also satisfy your taste buds.

Physical activity should be approached as a joyful expression of movement rather than a means of burning calories. Find activities that bring you joy, whether it's dancing, hiking, or practicing yoga. This shift in perspective transforms exercise from a chore into an integral part of your lifestyle.

Mindful practices, such as meditation and stress management, become essential components of this sustainable approach. Recognizing the interplay between mental and physical health is crucial for long-term success. It's not just about what you eat or how much you exercise; it's about cultivating a mindset that supports your overall well-being.

This shift is a process of self-discovery, exploring what truly works for your body and lifestyle. It's about creating a personalized, sustainable tapestry of choices that brings balance and fulfillment. As you embark on this journey, remember that it's not about perfection but progress—a continual evolution toward a healthier, happier you.

By embracing this shift from restrictive dieting to sustainable lifestyle choices, you empower yourself to make decisions that align with your long-term health goals. This approach is not a temporary fix but a commitment to a lifetime of well-being, creating a fulfilling and nourishing narrative for your unique journey.

Inspiring Others: Sharing Your Success Story

Sharing your success story is not just an act of personal celebration; it becomes a beacon of inspiration for others navigating their wellness journey. As you reflect on your achievements, consider the profound impact your story can have on fostering a supportive community and motivating others to embrace a healthier lifestyle.

Begin by acknowledging the unique path you've traveled—the challenges, triumphs, and gradual evolution toward a more balanced life. Your narrative is not just about weight loss or physical transformations; it encapsulates the holistic transformation of mind, body, and spirit.

Describe the pivotal moments that shaped your journey. Whether it was the decision to prioritize mental well-being, discovering the joy of nourishing meals, or finding fulfillment in physical activity, these moments became the building blocks of inspiration. Emphasize the small, consistent efforts that cumulatively led to significant changes.

Your success story isn't defined by rigid rules or perfection. Share the flexibility and adaptability that allowed you to overcome obstacles and setbacks. It's in these moments of resilience and determination that your story becomes relatable and encouraging for others facing similar challenges.

Highlight the role of a supportive community or the positive influence of mentors and resources that guided you along the way. Acknowledge that the journey is not solitary but a collective effort—a shared tapestry of experiences that connect individuals striving for better health.

Avoid presenting your journey as an unattainable feat but rather as a realistic and achievable transformation. Let readers understand that your success is rooted in choices that align with long-term well-being, emphasizing that anyone can embark on a similar path with commitment and self-compassion.

Encourage readers to celebrate their victories, no matter how small, and to view setbacks as opportunities for growth. Frame your story as an invitation for others to explore what works best for them, to experiment with different approaches, and to craft a wellness journey uniquely suited to their needs and preferences.

In inspiring others through your success story, you become a catalyst for positive change. Your narrative serves as a guidepost, shedding light on the possibilities within everyone's grasp. By sharing the genuine, human aspects of your journey, you contribute to a collective narrative of well-being, fostering a community where stories intertwine and individuals find motivation and encouragement to embrace a healthier, happier life.

Chapter 10

Resources for Continued Success

Embarking on a road toward sustainable health and well-being takes not only passion and devotion but also a smart approach to finding the correct resources. These materials operate as pillars, supporting your continuous success and giving you the tools necessary for continued growth and improvement.

An important resource on your route to success is knowledge. Stay informed on the newest breakthroughs in nutrition, exercise research, and mental well-being. Reputable websites, scientific publications, and books produced by professionals on the topic can serve as important references, ensuring that your decisions are rooted in evidence-based information.

Building a network of support is another crucial resource. Engage with like-minded individuals who have similar health and well-being goals. Social media platforms, online forums, and local community groups provide areas where you can share experiences, seek guidance, and take inspiration from the collective wisdom of others on similar journeys.

The world of wellness applications offers a wealth of tools at your fingertips. From meal planning and fitness monitoring to meditation and stress management, there are programs designed to help every facet of your well-being. Integrating these tools into your routine can streamline your efforts and provide guidance and incentives.

Professional guidance is an excellent resource that can help fine-tune your strategy. Nutritionists, personal trainers, and mental health professionals possess the competence to offer specialized recommendations targeted to your unique needs. Their support can help you overcome problems, optimize your methods, and guarantee that your trip remains pleasurable and sustainable.

Exploring various nutritious meals can strengthen your cooking skills and add to your long-term success. Cookbooks, cooking shows, and internet recipe platforms can inspire, turning meal preparation into a creative and pleasant component of your wellness regimen.

Prioritizing self-care routines is vital for sustaining a healthy and sustainable lifestyle. Incorporate activities that support your mental and emotional well-being, such as mindfulness, yoga, or nature walks. These techniques add to your overall resilience and guarantee that your journey is not only physically satisfying but also emotionally enjoyable.

Celebrating milestones and little successes is an often overlooked but crucial resource for continuing success. Acknowledge and appreciate the improvements you accomplish, no matter how tiny. This positive reinforcement builds motivation, turning your path into a succession of victories that propel you ahead.

In weaving these tools into the fabric of your wellness journey, you establish a foundation for continued success. Each resource performs a particular role, contributing to the strength of your approach. As you harness these tools, may your path be guided by wisdom, supported by community, and enriched by the understanding that you have the resources needed for a lifetime of well-being.

Recommended Books and Cookbooks

In the enormous world of health and wellness literature, discovering insightful and credible resources is vital for developing a strong foundation on your journey to well-being. Here are some highly recommended books and cookbooks that offer a lot of knowledge and inspiration:

"The Omnivore's Dilemma" by Michael Pollan:

Michael Pollan digs into the complexity of the current food system, analyzing the impact of our food choices on our health and the environment. His investigative approach enables readers to make informed judgments about what they eat.

"Atomic Habits" by James Clear:

James Clear's work provides a convincing foundation for understanding how habits impact our lives. This book is a useful resource for individuals seeking to make sustainable lifestyle changes, presenting practical ideas for creating beneficial habits.

"How Not to Die" by Michael Greger:

Dr. Michael Greger analyzes the link between diet and chronic diseases, giving evidence-based nutrition advice.

This thorough handbook empowers readers to make decisions that encourage longevity and general well-being.

"Salt, Fat, Acid, Heat" by Samin Nosrat:

Samin Nosrat's cookbook is a great resource for individuals wishing to better their culinary talents. Focusing on the essential aspects of cooking, the book empowers readers to produce delicious and well-balanced meals.

"Mindless Eating" by Brian Wansink:

Brian Wansink analyzes the psychology underlying our eating patterns, providing light on the elements that influence our food choices. This excellent book gives practical strategies for adopting a mindful approach to eating.

"The Plant Paradox" by Steven R. Gundry:

Dr. Gundry questions conventional dietary thinking, studying the function of specific plant-based foods in human health. The book provides an alternate perspective on nutrition and offers tips on developing a balanced and satisfying diet.

" Titled: The Joy of Cooking" by Irma S. Rombauer:

A classic in the culinary world, this cookbook is a timeless resource for both beginners and seasoned cooks. With a wide choice of recipes and culinary suggestions, it develops a love for making healthy and delicious meals.

"Eat, Pray, Love" by Elizabeth Gilbert:

While not a standard health book, Elizabeth Gilbert's voyage of self-discovery, including her research of food in Italy, gives a refreshing take on the connection between enjoyment, sustenance, and overall well-being.

These recommended books and cookbooks serve as essential companions on your journey for a better and more fulfilling existence. Each one adds a distinct perspective, providing the knowledge and inspiration needed to make educated decisions and adopt a well-rounded approach to well-being.

Online Communities for Support

In the digital era, the pursuit of a healthier lifestyle should not be a solo trip. The development of Internet networks has provided individuals with virtual support, information, and fellowship while they pursue their wellness goals. These groups, anchored in the shared principles of health and self-improvement, offer a plethora of resources to sweeten the reader's pursuit of a healthy and full life.

1. Reddit's r/HealthyLiving Community: The broad Reddit platform contains a plethora of health-related communities, with r/HealthyLiving being a hub for different conversations. From nutrition suggestions to fitness routines, this community provides an open environment where individuals share stories and advice, creating a supportive environment for people on their wellness journey.

2. My Fitness Pal's Community Forums: MyFitnessPal, a popular program for tracking nutrition and activity, expands its help beyond data submission. The app's community forums provide a venue for users to share triumphs, seek advice, and engage in debates about health and well-being. This virtual tapestry of experiences gives motivation and direction to people negotiating the intricacies of healthier living.

3. SparkPeople's Team Forums: SparkPeople, a holistic wellness platform, promotes the significance of community through its team forums. These forums cover a wide range of topics, from fitness challenges to recipe exchanges, weaving a vibrant tapestry of encouragement and connection among individuals aiming for improved health.

4. Fitbit Community: Fitbit, recognized for its activity monitors, claims a robust online community where users can share successes, set challenges, and seek help. This platform weaves together a tapestry of fitness aficionados, providing a sense of friendship that transcends regional bounds.

5. Instagram's Health and Well-Being Hashtags: The visual appeal of Instagram extends into the area of health and happiness, with numerous hashtags like HealthyLiving and WellnessJourney. Users can explore this virtual tapestry of curated content, receiving inspiration from others' healthy meals, workout regimens, and mindful living habits.

6. Facebook Groups for Wellbeing: Facebook, a platform connecting billions globally, hosts various groups dedicated to wellbeing. Whether focused on specific diets, fitness routines, or overall well-being, these organizations create a digital tapestry of shared experiences, fostering a sense of community among members.

7. Health Blogs and Forums:

Numerous health-focused blogs and forums, such as HealthBoards and WebMD's community, provide areas for users to share health-related insights, seek advice, and offer encouragement. These platforms contribute to a wide tapestry of knowledge, experiences, and stories that appeal to readers.

In the world of online communities, individuals might find a supportive tapestry that corresponds with their wellness aspirations. As readers connect with these digital forums, they get knit into a fabric of shared experiences, various opinions, and mutual encouragement—creating a dynamic and enriching environment to support their journey toward a healthier and more balanced existence.

Tools and Apps for Tracking Progress

In the pursuit of a better lifestyle, the integration of current technologies and software has altered the way individuals track and assess their progress. These digital companions serve as important resources, bringing insights, motivation, and a streamlined approach to well-being.

1. MyFitnessPal: MyFitnessPal stands as a stalwart in the area of health apps, providing a comprehensive platform for tracking both nutrition and exercise. Users may effortlessly register meals, set fitness goals, and analyze their progress over time. The app's huge database streamlines the process of recording food intake, adding to a seamless and successful tracking experience.

2. Fitbit: Fitbit, synonymous with activity monitoring, offers a suite of gadgets and simple software to measure physical activity, sleep habits, and general wellness. With features like heart rate monitoring and personalized insights, Fitbit converts the tracking journey into a visually appealing and informative experience, encouraging customers to stay engaged with their health goals.

3. Apple Health: Integrated into Apple products, Apple Health acts as a consolidated hub for health and fitness data.

This program smoothly collates information from multiple sources, such as fitness apps, wearable devices, and manual inputs. Its user-friendly interface gives a clear summary of one's health parameters, creating a sense of control and awareness.

4. Google Fit: For Android users, Google Fit emerges as a powerful platform for activity tracking and health monitoring. This app leverages the sensors in smartphones and wearables to record statistics on steps walked, calories burnt, and heart rate. The intuitive design helps consumers to keep informed about their daily exercise levels.

5. Cronometer: Cronometer specializes in rigorous nutritional tracking, delivering a comprehensive breakdown of micronutrients with macronutrients. This software provides a deeper understanding of dietary choices, ensuring that users maintain a balanced and nutrient-rich diet. With its emphasis on nutritional fullness, Cronometer contributes to a holistic monitoring experience.

6. HabitBull: Recognizing the importance of creating positive habits, HabitBull gets into the arena with a focus on habit formation and consistency. Users can measure activities such as hydration, frequent exercise, or mindful eating. The app's visual portrayal of streaks and awards transforms the tracking procedure into a gratifying and encouraging trip.

7. Strava: For fitness aficionados, Strava acts as a dedicated program for recording running and cycling activities. It not only analyzes performance indicators but also develops a sense of community by allowing users to share their successes and participate in challenges. The communal aspect adds a degree of motivation, turning the tracking experience into a shared undertaking.

Incorporating these tools and apps into one's wellness journey increases the tracking process, making it more accessible, entertaining, and instructive. By using the power of technology, individuals may effortlessly weave progress monitoring into their daily lives, producing a rich and dynamic tapestry of data that reflects their journey toward optimal health and well-being.

Conclusion

As we draw the curtains on this balanced and thoughtful approach to nourishing the body, it's obvious that the journey toward wellness is not a solitary path but a tapestry woven from diverse threads of information, decisions, and experiences. We've traveled the realms of nutrition, indulgence, mindful eating, and the psychology underlying our culinary choices, all with the overriding purpose of encouraging a healthier, more balanced existence.

In the feast of life, our connection with food plays a key role, determining not only our bodily well-being but also our mental and emotional states. From grasping the relevance of macronutrients in extravagant eating to embracing mindful tactics and designing delicious meals, every choice becomes a brushstroke in the canvas of our health.

We've studied the art of leisurely eating, the significance of designing a balanced plate, and the impact of flavor on our satisfaction and satiety. By connecting with our hunger and fullness cues and adopting mindful food choices, we begin a journey of self-discovery and self-care.

The psychology of excess has been unwrapped, showing the delicate dance between our desires and our well-being. Breaking free from guilt and food shame becomes a vital step toward building a healthy relationship with the food we consume, nurturing an environment where occasional indulgence is not only allowed but appreciated.

Through the chapters that emerged, we've uncovered the relevance of portion management without deprivation, the joy of constructing meals for optimum flavor and satisfaction, and the importance of pampering oneself without derailing the pursuit of health. Culinary inventiveness, from savory breakfasts to indulgent feasts, has been studied as a technique to transform our meals into moments of great enjoyment.

We've handled the hurdles of dining out, mingling, and celebrating without compromising our goals, learning how to make indulgent choices in varied settings. Fitness and fun have been interwoven, highlighting the balance between action and excess. The role of exercise in a balanced lifestyle has been stressed, concentrating not just on the physical benefits but the mental and emotional pleasures as well.

In addressing frequent challenges, overcoming emotional eating, handling plateaus and failures, and staying motivated for long-term success, we've discovered that resilience is a critical element in our formula for enduring well-being. By embracing the journey and celebrating tiny accomplishments, we shift from dieting to sustainable lifestyle choices, establishing a tapestry of habits that survive the test of time.

The resources for continuous success, whether in the shape of recommended books and cookbooks or online groups for support, serve as pillars that sustain our commitment to a better lifestyle. Tracking progress through tools and apps becomes a natural part of our routine, delivering insights and inspiration to keep us on track.

As we complete this educational journey, remember that each step you take towards a better living is a win. Your decisions count, and the devotion you've shown to your well-being is a monument to your strength. May your road be paved with happiness, fulfillment, and a great sense of success. Here's to your continuing success on this journey toward a balanced and nutritious existence.

Recap of Key Principles

In the process of building a balanced and thoughtful lifestyle, we have found essential principles that act as guiding stars on the way to well-being. These concepts encompass the essence of maintaining a balanced connection with food, exercise, and the road toward sustained health.

First and foremost, the necessity of mindful eating strategies has been underlined. By paying intentional attention to the sensory experience of eating, from the flavors to the textures, we boost our satisfaction and satiety. This awareness extends to identifying hunger and fullness cues, ensuring that our bodies receive the food they need without excess.

The art of leisurely eating arose as a crucial method for appreciating our meals. By allowing ourselves the time to appreciate each bite, we not only boost the pleasure of eating but also enable our bodies to communicate fullness more correctly. Slow eating converts our meals into moments of enjoyment rather than mere replenishment.

Building a balanced plate has been a repeated theme, highlighting the need to integrate a variety of colorful and nutrient-dense meals. This not only ensures a varied variety of critical nutrients but also adds brightness and taste to our meals. Portion restriction without deprivation has been proposed as a sustainable method, noting that satisfaction need not be lost for health.

Mindful dietary choices have been identified as essential drivers to long-term satisfaction. By making intentional judgments about what we consume, we empower ourselves to connect our dietary habits with our health goals. This method surpasses mere limitations, building a good and meaningful relationship with the foods we choose to include in our diet.

The research on the psychology of indulgence delved into the complicated interplay between our desires, emotions, and well-being. Breaking free from guilt and food shame appeared as a transforming step toward having a happy connection with food. By enjoying occasional excess and indulging ourselves without deprivation, we remove the restricted mindset frequently linked with good eating.

Crafting meals for optimal flavor and happiness became a cornerstone of our culinary journey. Incorporating bright and nutrient-dense items further boosts the visual appeal and nutritious value of our dishes. The ideas of portion control, conscious decisions, and indulgence in moderation contribute to a balanced and satisfying approach to feeding.

Fitness, as a vital aspect of a balanced lifestyle, has been stressed not just for its physical benefits but also for the joy and excitement it gives. The function of exercise in a balanced lifestyle extends beyond calorie expenditure, embracing mental and emotional well-being.

In managing challenges, overcoming emotional eating, and staying motivated for long-term success, resilience emerged as a defining attribute. By embracing the process and appreciating tiny accomplishments, we shift from dieting to sustainable lifestyle choices. The resources for continuous success, from recommended books and cookbooks to online groups and tracking tools, serve as helpful companions on this ongoing path to well-being.

In this brief, we've touched upon the key concepts that form the cornerstone of balanced and thoughtful living. Each concept, when embraced, leads to a harmonious and sustainable approach to health. As you integrate these ideas into your daily life, may they guide you toward a future filled with vitality, satisfaction, and enduring well-being.

Your Personalized Path to Indulgent, Nourishing Eating

Embarking on your route to rich, nourishing eating is a process of self-discovery and conscious decisions. As you travel this route, it's vital to remember that there's no one-size-fits-all approach to healthy living. Instead, it's about building an eating experience that corresponds with your particular preferences, requirements, and goals.

Begin by tuning into your body's messages. Understanding your hunger and fullness cues creates the cornerstone of a personalized strategy. By paying attention to when your body indicates hunger and when it conveys fullness, you empower yourself to make choices that honor your body's natural rhythms.

Consider the flavors and textures that excite your palate. Every individual has a particular taste profile, and embracing the foods you appreciate ensures that your meals are a source of enjoyment. Whether it's the crispness of fresh veggies, the richness of particular proteins, or the sweetness of fruits, let your personal preferences dictate your culinary selections.

Building a balanced dish tailored to your dietary needs is crucial. This involves incorporating a variety of colorful and nutrient-dense foods. Think of your plate as a canvas where you paint with a diversity of vegetables, lean proteins, complete grains, and healthy fats. This not only supplies critical nutrients but also adds visual appeal and different flavors to your meals.

Mindful meal choices play a significant role in personalizing your eating journey. Consider the source, quality, and nutritional worth of the meals you consume. Opting for whole, minimally processed foods ensures that your body receives the nourishment it needs. Mindfulness extends beyond the act of eating — it's about building a conscious awareness of the complete food experience, from purchasing to preparation and consumption.

Portion control remains an important part of individualized eating. Understanding the proper portion sizes for your unique needs minimizes overeating and allows you to enjoy your favorite meals in moderation. This technique removes the concept of deprivation, promoting a good relationship with food.

Indulgence, in moderation, is a necessary component of your particular path. Treating yourself occasionally to meals you appreciate leads to a balanced and happy eating experience. This is not about guilt or shame but about relishing the flavors and building a healthy relationship with occasional pleasures.

Crafting meals for optimal flavor and satisfaction fits with your specific preferences. Whether you love robust and spicy flavors or enjoy experimenting with herbs and spices, your culinary selections should provide delight and fulfillment. The psychology of indulgence, when understood and managed properly, becomes a strong instrument in your individualized strategy.

Your journey to individualized, enjoyable, and satisfying eating is a dynamic and continuous process. It's about understanding what works best for you and adapting as your needs change. As you accept this path, may it be one filled with delight, satisfaction, and a profound connection to the sustenance your body deserves.